Your Health

It's a Question of Balance

About the Authors

Doctor Igor Cetojevic was born in Bugojno, Bosnia-Herzegovina. After completing his medical degree in Sarajevo in 1988, he studied Chinese Traditional Medicine. Since 2001, he specializes in biofeedback therapy and health education, often working with top-class athletes.

See: www.DrIgor.org

Francesca Pinoni was born in San Francisco, California. She earned a BA in Theatre Arts form the University of California at Santa Cruz. Since 1994 she has been working closely with Igor to develop his work and communicate it to a broader audience and working to promote the acceptance of complementary therapies in Cyprus.

Your Health

It's a Question of Balance

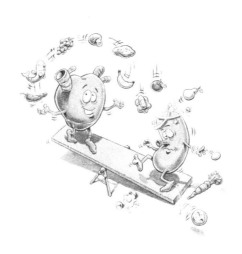

Dr. Igor Cetojevic

& Francesca Pinoni

Cover art and interior illustrations by Jim Caputo

Revised Edition 2014

ISBN: 978-9963-9651-4-4
Featherlight Press
P.O. Box 51958, 3509 Limassol. Cyprus
featherlight@cyprusspirit.com

For our friends

Dedication

We would like to dedicate this book, first of all, to each other with love. Through the process of writing it we experienced a dynamic balance of our strengths and weaknesses, and, hopefully produced something greater than the sum of our individual parts.

Secondly, to our friends in Cyprus, the island of love, who offered us their hands, hearths and hearts. Thirdly, we dedicate it to you, the reader. Without you we might as well be talking to ourselves. We hope that between these covers you'll find some small gems to keep in your pocket and bring a smile to your face; a few simple truths that can make a big difference when put into practice.

Special thanks to Alex Toumazis for his invaluable help with the computer and patience regarding meal times.

This book not is intended as a replacement for good medical diagnosis. It is written for educational purposes as a means to help people to make informed choices about their health and lifestyle options.

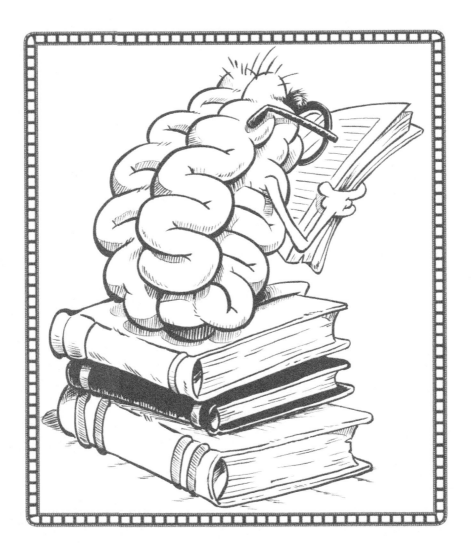

Contents

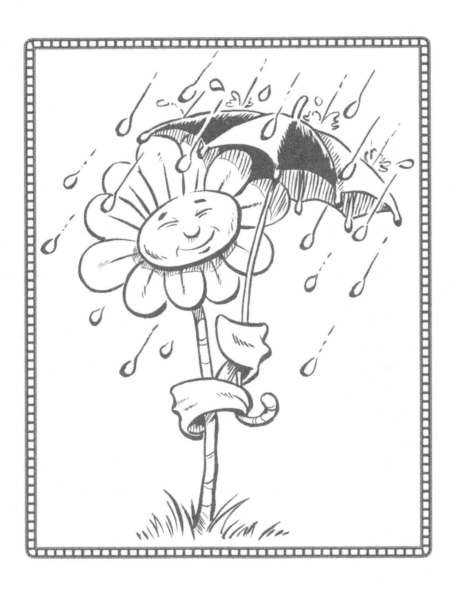

Welcome

I met Igor at my son's eighth birthday party, which was at my house. A mutual friend brought him along. After the cake and ice cream, Igor showed the children how a pendulum works. They were spell bound, as was I. As people were leaving I went over to Igor and asked, "Can you teach me to do that?" "Yes I can," he said, and so began the road, long, full of pot holes, roundabouts and a lot of fun that has led to our eventual marriage and the writing of this book.

In the early days of our friendship (and my apprenticeship) I had to pay really close attention to what Igor was telling me because his English, as he would say, "Is not so good." I carried around a little blue notebook with "Notes from Dr. Igor" written on the front cover. So many interesting things would come up in the normal course of our conversations that I decided to take notes. My little blue notebook became the basis for this book.

I grew up in California and had always been health conscious. I watched what I ate and knew the importance of exercise. Although I knew that diet was important, I didn't really understand why, nor did I comprehend how the body works. I had never heard about the negative effects that underground and electromagnetic vibrations have on our health. Everything that Igor told me had such a lovely simplicity and feeling of truth to it. I was hooked.

He explained, very simply, how energy works, how the different organs in the body work and how simple it is to stay healthy if you know how - and are prepared to take responsibility for your own health. I followed his advice and feel healthier now than I have ever felt in my life. I've watched other people follow his advice and make dramatic improvements in their health and happiness.

It is with this insight and passion that we would like to share this information to you.

Francesca Pinoni

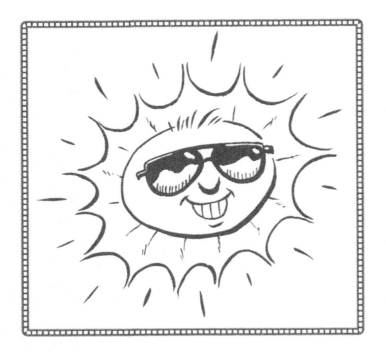

Introduction

I would like to explain my strategy of healing. I qualified as a Medical Doctor, General Practitioner. When I completed my studies and started to practice medicine I found that something was missing. Although I had been trained well and had good knowledge of Western medicine I felt that it did not provide enough information to effectively heal my patients. It wasn't enough to prescribe medicine to patients and send them off to wait and see if it worked or not; a practice that seemed to me to be the essence of Western medicine. Sometimes it worked and sometimes it didn't, and when it didn't then another medicine would be tried. It seemed like a lot of trial and error. The patients would be lucky if the side effects of the "cure" were less uncomfortable than their original condition. What effect does this have on the physical and mental health of the patient?

Thank goodness I had the opportunity to learn about Chinese Traditional Medicine and acupuncture. I studied Traditional Chinese Medicine and acupuncture for two years in Belgrade, Yugoslavia, followed by advanced courses in Beijing, China. From those studies, I learned how to look at a patient's problem from a totally different perspective.

I learned about a "whole-system" philosophy that takes into account the entire person rather than a system that views the body as a machine and attempts to fix its individual parts. Chinese medicine focuses on identifying and treating the *root cause* of a problem rather than by merely alleviating the symptoms. This process sometimes takes a little longer but, in the long run, proves to be a much more efficient method of treatment. Once the root cause has been eliminated a person will remain healthy. When only the symptom is treated, the problem will resurface either as the same condition or a different one based on the same root cause.

One education gave me one body of information; the other education gave me another one, but even with all this information I knew something was missing. As a child I would drive my parents crazy by always asking, "Why" and "What?" over and over again. I guess it is this insatiable curiosity that prompts me to always be on the lookout for more information, more knowledge and more pieces of the puzzle that will eventually add up to maximum health.

One day while I was studying in Beijing, China, I was sitting at the lunch table with a Chinese doctor. We talked about the difference between Chinese and Western medicine. He pointed to a teapot on the table between us and said, "Look at that teapot...tell me about it." I said, "It's white, it has a spout to pour the tea." "Anything else?" he asked me. "No." "What about the pink flower?" He turned the teapot around and I saw that there was a flower painted on that side. "If we look at things from different ways, we can observe different things. We could argue for hours about whether the tea pot was plain white or if it had a flower on it. We are both right, from our individual perspectives. But look how much more we know when we share out observations and our points of view."

After studying both Western and Eastern healing systems, I encountered a very special doctor while attending a seminar in Belgrade. His name was Dr. Nikola Videv and he showed me, for the first time in my life, the etheric body. We covered many topics in Dr. Videv's class: acupuncture meridians, energy, chi, the Tao, AURA, the etheric body - lots of interesting material. During one of the classes he gave us some information about vibrational medicine and dowsing. That was the first time that I heard about these things. I'd seen people fooling around with pendulums but I always thought it was silly. This time, however, I had a strong feeling that this information was something that would play an important role in my life.

I was impressed that a respected doctor in his mid-fifties, whose specialty was psychiatry, would stand up in front of a group of advanced students, all qualified doctors, many of them over fifty years old, and talk to us about such things as dowsing and vibrational medicine. It's often difficult for medical doctors to open doors and windows to let in fresh air from a different direction.

Dr. Videv stood in front of the class and said, "Dear friends, I will show you something that would be very interesting for you to practice." He showed us two ordinary metal rods about eighteen inches long bent at right angles like an L. With his elbows near the sides of his body, he held the rods so that they were parallel to the floor. Then he walked across the classroom and something happened. At certain spots in the room the ends of the rods came together. As he kept walking they separated again. Why was that happening? Was the doctor moving the rods? If so, why? What's going on here? Again… why and what!

Then he took out a chain with a small metal cone attached: a pendulum. He put one hand on his heart and held the chain of the pendulum between the thumb and index finger of his other hand. Again he walked around the room. In some places the pendulum spun around in a circle. In other places it stopped moving. Why?

Dr. Vedev explained that he was using the L-rods and pendulum as tools to make the unseen vibrations in the environment visible. He went on to tell us the effect that these vibrations have on our health and the health of our patients. This information touched me deeply and I would now like to share it with you. Neither Western nor Eastern medicine takes into consideration the influence of vibrations around us when looking into a patient's condition. These disturbing vibrations are caused by natural conditions in the earth or by man-made electrical equipment.

He shared how he observed this influence in the course of his work in a psychiatric hospital. "I was working in a hospital and had the idea to check the vibrations in the location of my patients' beds. One bed was in a spot that had a particularly harmful vibrational influence. I observed that patients who were in that particular bed suffered more acute symptoms than his neighbors in the ward who had similar complaints and were on similar medication. When these patients were moved to another bed, their condition immediately improved." Dr. Videv explained that people with psychiatric problems are more sensitive to vibrations around them; their threshold of sensitivity is higher than average. For example, even when a light is switched on near them they react more strongly than we would. Being in a place of strong negative vibration is like a slap to them.

Dr. Videv told us, "It is difficult to explain this briefly, but if some of you practice yoga or mediation you may find it easier to use these tools." His words touched me again because I was interested in both yoga and meditation. I was sitting in the front row and eagerly volunteered to try the tools that he had shown us. He explained that for the tools to work we must keep our minds out of the picture and not expect anything to happen. I took the rods and walked across the room. I felt them moving in my hands! I knew that I had not consciously moved them and felt exhilaration because, yes, I could actually do this. Dr. Videv looked me in the eye and said, "I think you are a good receiver. It is necessary for you to start slowly and check many places. You need years to be sure you know what you are doing." Now, after many years of checking space and people I am sure of what I am doing! And I would like to offer my knowledge to you.

What did I do with the information I learned from Dr. Videv? I applied his methods to my own system of treating patients by using acupuncture and herbs. As a result, their energy levels increased. Sometimes patients would respond well to treatment, but the next day their energy would drop and they would feel unwell again. I compare the body to a rechargeable battery: during the treatment the battery fills up with energy; however, something causes the battery to leak energy. I knew my patient was following my instructions regarding proper food and medicinal herbs, so what was the problem? Why wasn't the patient getting better? Again why and what? I remembered Dr. Videv's lecture and decided to check the places where my patients spent a lot of time - the places where they slept and the places where they worked. Invariably, the patients who were not retaining the energy that was built up during their treatments were spending considerable time in places with strong negative vibrational influences. When they moved their beds or desks to a better position, their condition improved dramatically. They no longer lost the energy they acquired and they were able to add more energy with each additional treatment.

My mother was a teacher. Once I went to visit her at school. During recess, I checked her classroom and found one particularly bad spot. Without letting on why I wanted to know I asked, "Mom, who sits here?" "Oh", she said, "One very naughty boy. He can never sit still. He's always on the edge of his chair." Obviously, he was trying to get away from that spot with disturbing vibrations. I asked her to move his desk to another spot. She did, and as if by magic, his behavior changed. He was less restless and his concentration improved. Children have strong instincts, like animals. They are open. They like something or they don't. They do not like places with disturbing vibrations and do whatever they can to get away from them.

On another occasion I was treating a woman at her home in Belgrade. It was difficult for her to relax during her treatment because her twin infant daughters would not stop crying. When I asked her why they cried so much she said she didn't know; she had taken them to several doctors and was told that there was nothing wrong with them. The family was happy and economically stable. There was no apparent reason for the babies to cry so much. I asked her to show me where they slept. When I checked the room I found that both their cribs were in very bad spots. I noticed that one of the cribs had an unusually high side and asked their mother about it. She said, "My baby kept rolling off the bed. We had to make the side higher to keep her in. The other baby sleeps huddled up in the corner of her crib." I advised the mother to move the cribs to the other side of the room out of the areas that had strong vibrations. She agreed and we moved them together, there and then. The following week I went to her home again to treat her. She looked much better and was much more relaxed. I had hardly walked through the door when she told me, "My neighbor came by yesterday and asked me, "Where are your babies?" They have been so quiet since we moved their beds that the neighbors thought they weren't here anymore!"

Since then I have observed time and time again that by locating the places of negative vibrational influence and repositioning the furniture so that one does not spend a lot of time in there, many chronic symptoms disappear.

I also use the pendulum to check the energy of my patients. The pendulum is my "x-ray". It shows me where the patient's weaknesses are and how they are responding to treatment. When I check a patient, I use a lot of synonyms for what I am measuring: temperature, bio-energy, etheric body and aura. This is nothing new. Some people can see the human aura. I can feel it.

It is important for my patients to know that I am a medical doctor and that I have gained a lot of knowledge from both Western and Eastern medical traditions. When a patient comes to see me I tell him or her, "You are not my patient, you are my friend. I ask you to take *responsibility* for your body, mind and spirit. Using all my knowledge, I will do all my best to help you. But, in the end, it is your body and your responsibility to take care of it. There is a big problem today with people not taking responsibility for themselves. Some people expect their physicians to "fix" them when they become ill. They seem to have the attitude that they can eat all the rubbish they see advertised on television, smoke, lead an inactive life, and when they get sick the insurance company will cover the cost of making them better. If they don't get better, they often blame the doctors, because, after all, they are being paid to cure them. Well, it doesn't work that way.

I liken my view of healing to this sign:

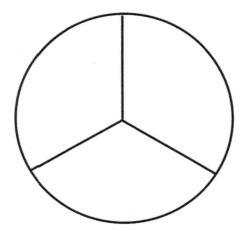

If I use all my knowledge, do all my best work; the maximum I can contribute is one third of the whole picture:

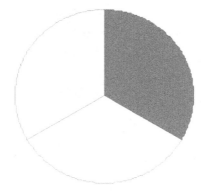

If my patients follows my recommendations and take responsibility for their own healing process, then add another third.

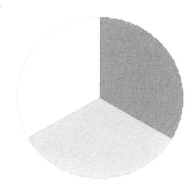

Two thirds is more than half way there. Our combined human effort in coming this far invites help from a higher power. The last third is in the hands of God.

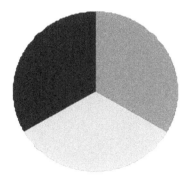

I would like to teach people how to take responsibility for their third. In this book I will explain a simple way of understanding what it takes to create your own health. I'll show you the pieces of the puzzle that, when gathered together, can create total health. It's really very simple - when you know how. And that's what this book is about.

Let's go!

1   In the Beginning

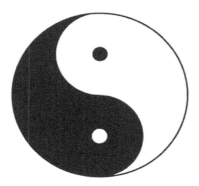

You've seen this sign, a black and white circle like two fish swimming head to tail. Do you know what it means?

For our purpose, let's call this the Yin / Yang Sign. It is the basis of understanding *dynamic balance*, and balance is the key to health. Pretty simple so far.

All things in this world can be viewed as either Yin or Yang, two opposite things that cannot exist without each other. The shape of the sign signifies both unity and motion. Nothing is static. What is Yin now is moving towards becoming Yang, and what is Yang now is moving towards becoming Yin. You say, "This isn't so simple..."

But, here's an example: Think of a year starting from the middle of winter. This is as Yin as it gets. It's cold, its dark, the days are short and the nights are long. As the months pass, soon it is springtime. At the time of the spring equinox the lengths of the day and the night are the same. The temperatures are mild, neither hot nor cold. There is a moment of perfect equilibrium, and then what happens? There is a shift to the Yang side. The days become hotter and longer until midsummer. What happens then? Does it get hotter and hotter? No, the balance starts to shift again as fall follows summer with another moment of equilibrium until Yin begins to predominate again. And so it goes, over and over again, year in and year out.

So what? First, you can see that the ratio of Yin to Yang changes as the earth moves through her seasonal changes, and this cycle repeats itself indefinitely. Second, you have learned some of the properties of Yin (cold, dark) and Yang (hot, light). Third, a state of balance is not static, everything moves and changes and still preserves its balance. Fourth, and a little more subtly, you may have realized that the varying amount of Yin and Yang through the course of the year might just have an effect on our health.

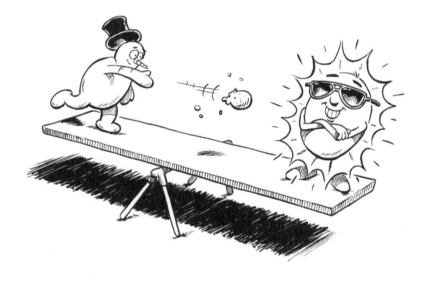

I'll be using this seesaw a lot. It illustrates pretty clearly the idea of dynamic balance.

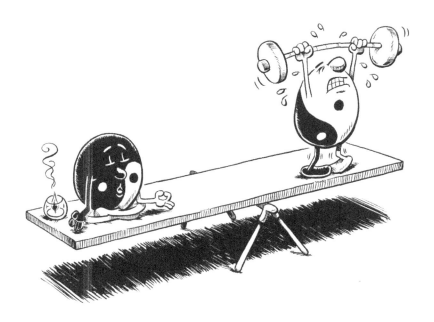

Yin and Yang are foreign words. Think of Yin as being a magnetic or contracting force (like gravity, something that pulls something into itself) and Yang as being a dynamic or expanding force (like centrifugal force, which is what you see in a clothes dryer; it's the force that pushes things away from itself).

Take a moment to observe yourself. How are you sitting right now? You can learn a lot from your body.

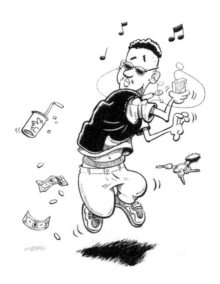

This is a Yang position.

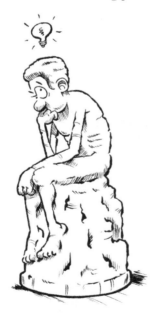

This is a Yin position.

How come and what does it mean? I'll explain.

Here are some attributes of Yin and Yang:

YIN	**YANG**
Feminine	Masculine
Cold	Hot
Wet	Dry
Closing	Opening
Contraction	Expansion
Stillness	Movement
Dark	Light
Magnetic	Dynamic
Sweet	Salty

Salty? Sweet? What's this? Well, I'm sneaking in something important here.

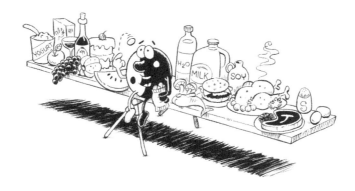

Let's take a look at food. We need food to live. We need food to get the vitamins, minerals, proteins, carbohydrates and fats that we need to energize and build our bodies. We need the *right* food to be healthy. You may be asking. "Why is he giving us information that is just common sense?" I know… you know these things already. But *what is the right food?*

There is no right food. Wait! Don't stone me yet! There is "right food" but it is not the same right food for everybody, at all times. Remember what I said right at the start of this chapter: Balance is the key.

Probably, you were taught from an early age that maintaining a balanced diet and eating nutritious food is good for you. Well, that is a good start. What is a balanced meal? It is considered to consist of foods from the different food groups, starches, meat, fruit and vegetables, and so forth. But this is not enough in itself. This simplified formula does not take into consideration other important factors such as the type of work you do, the climate in which you live, or the weather, for example.

I can hear you now. "You said this would be *simple* but if we have to think about all these things it won't be simple at all." Before you give up, slow down and keep reading.

Let's go back to our illustration of the seesaw:

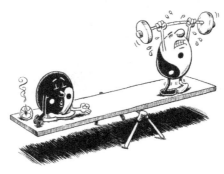

Here is the seesaw showing Yin and Yang as the extreme points. Our aim it to keep our balance.

When it is time to eat there are certain things to consider with a view toward this seesaw. They are:

- the relative position of the weather
- the relative position of the type of work that you are doing
- the relative position of the food on the seesaw

That's not so much, now, is it?

Let's start with the weather since you all know whether or not it's cold outside. Here's the seesaw: Hot is on the Yang side, cold is on the Yin side.

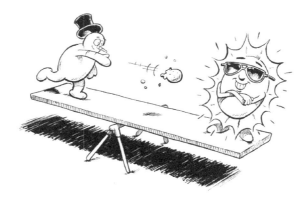

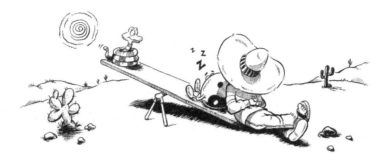

This is a very hot summer day in Mexico

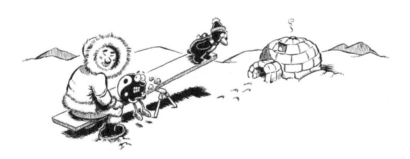

This is a snowy winter day in Alaska.

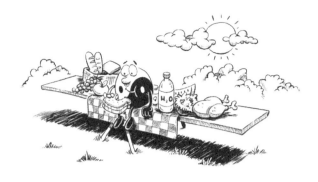

And this is a lovely day for a picnic.

Next let's look at the work we do. Some of us have jobs that require hard physical labor, erecting buildings, digging trenches, plowing the land, herding the cows; but most of us have pretty sedentary jobs these days.

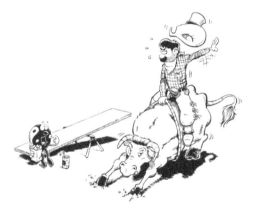

Here's a Cowboy. Being a cowboy required lots of activity.– Physical work depleted his Yang energy and he needs more Yang food to make the seesaw balance

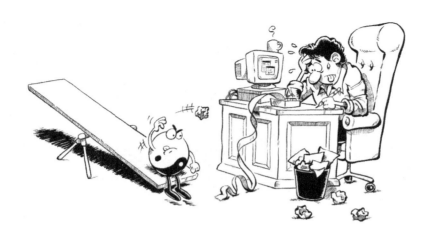

Here's an accountant. Being an accountant requires lots of brainwork. Mental work depleted his Yin energy and he needs more Yin food to balance the seesaw.

Do you find it easy to go outside and have a heavy workout on a very hot day? No way. Why? Because these is too much Yang in that equation. You literally burn up. Is it a coincidence that people who live in hot countries often take a siesta in the afternoon? I don't think so.

Now we come to food. This one is a little less obvious for those of us who grew up in the Western world. No one ever told us that some foods are Yin and others are Yang... Stay with me. You learned to count calories. This is a whole lot easier.

To put it simply, if a food is salty it is Yang. If it is sweet it is Yin. Here's a list starting with foods that are closest to the center of the seesaw.

Yin	Yang
Grains	Milk
Cereal	Mushrooms
Seeds (sesame, sunflower)	Beans
Yogurt	Soy Products
Oil (from seeds)	Cheese
Vegetables	Chicken
Garlic	Olive Oil
Fruit	Fish
Fruit Juice	Nuts
Sweets	Beef
Vinegar	Pork
Alcohol	Eggs
White Sugar	Salt

Generally speaking, salt is extreme Yang, proteins (such as red meat), are strong Yang; Fats are moderate Yang. Carbohydrates like grains and cereals, are moderate Yin, vitamins and minerals are Yin, and sweets are strong Yin, and white sugar is Yin to the max.

With a little practice, you can use a pendulum to test whether food is Yin or Yang. If you don't happen to have a ready-made pendulum lying around the house a key or a ring tied on a piece of string about five inches long works just fine. Practice first with unmarked salt and sugar.

Sit comfortably at your dining table. Have ready two identical bowls one with a tablespoon of sugar in it and another with a tablespoon of salt. Put your elbow on the table and hold the chain of the pendulum between your thumb and index finger. Hold it over the bowl containing the sugar and observe the movement of the pendulum. Relax your shoulders, elbows and wrists, and be patient. Keep breathing. Next, hold the pendulum over the salt. After a while, you should observe a different movement. Make a note of the direction the pendulum moves for sugar (Yin) and salt (Yang). The movements are not the same for everyone so you'll need to do this test first.

Just for fun, have someone change the position of the bowls so you don't know which one is which. Test the two bowls again and then check and see if you identified them correctly. If not, try again. And don't forget to breathe. This doesn't work if you hold your breath. Remember to be patient, as this can take some practice.

Once you and your pendulum can identify the sugar and salt, then you are ready to check other foods to see if they produce Yin or Yang energy.

Not all foods are created equal. Here is our friendly seesaw showing the relative positions of different Yin and Yang foods. As you get proficient with the pendulum, it will make bigger movements for foods that are close to the extremes.

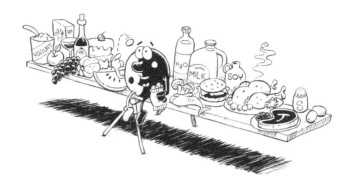

Rice and grains are just about in the center. These are balanced foods and combine well with other foods. Spring water is as good as it gets. Water helps balance the foods you eat. Have you noticed that when you eat very salty food or very sweet food you feel very thirsty? Now you know why. You body as asking for *balance.*

The idea is to create a meal that will perfectly balance the seesaw. You may think that you can do that by eating only brown rice (remember the macrobiotic diet?), but it doesn't quite work that way.

Some of you might be thinking, "Oh good. If I drink whiskey with my spareribs I'll have a perfect balance." Not quite. If you try to make a balance from *extreme* Yin and Yang it doesn't work. Imagine a heavy weight on either end of a seesaw. What happens? The seesaw breaks in two! *Crack*!!

The rice-only diet doesn't work unless you live in a perfect climate all year 'round, you do just enough mental and physical work and you don't have any stress or emotional ups and downs. Why? Because now it's time to put everything together on that handy little seesaw.

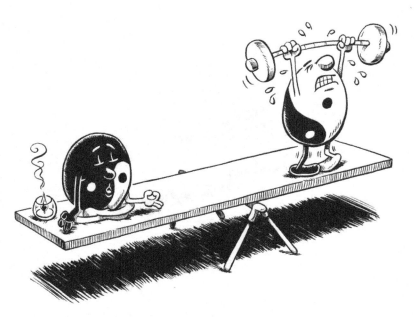

The starting point.

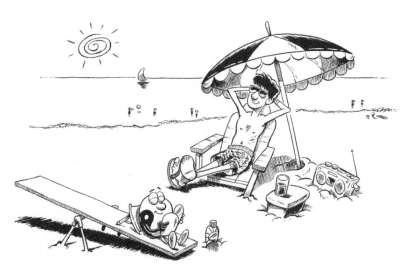

It's summer. It's a hot day...

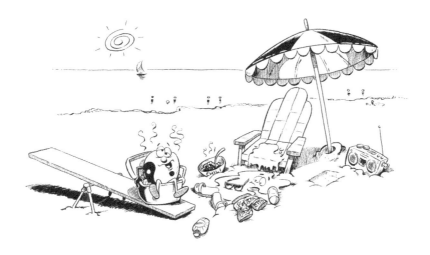

Add a bowl of chili and we hit bottom.

Way too Yang. So what do you do?

You go to sleep - an extreme Yin activity.

If you wanted to enjoy the rest of your day having fun at the beach instead of fast asleep in your bed, a more balanced meal would be a fresh salad and iced tea.

Bon appétit!

Now, close your eyes and try to imagine a vegetarian Eskimo. Too Yin. How about a South Sea Islander chomping on spare ribs and stew. It just does not compute.

Pretty simple, isn't it?

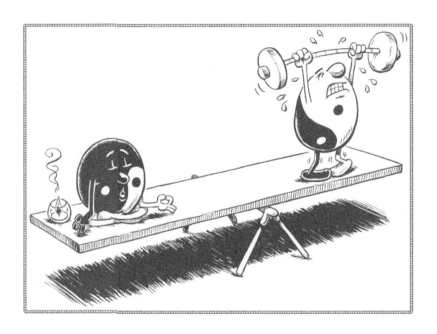

2 Ups and Downs

I started this book with an example of the yearly cycle. Now I will show you more about how the different cycles of the year and even of each day provide clues that will help you to keep yourself in top shape.

First let me give you a little lesson:

Chinese Medicine 1A

All our organs are either Yin or Yang. How can you tell which is which? It's pretty easy. The Yin organs are generally compact and more solid and the Yang organs are hollow like bags that let things flow through them.

Every organ has a buddy. They make a co-operative couple; one Yin organ with one Yang organ. Each pair of organs is associated with an opening in your face. So, be aware that you are showing your state of health to anyone who knows where to look. Pretty soon you will know where to look, too.

Each pair of organs is also associated with an emotion. Emotion! What do emotions have to do with the physical body? Plenty - as we will see later.

Each season of the year is associated with one pair of organs.

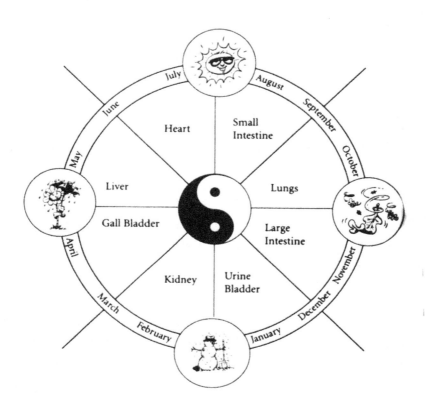

As you can see, each pair of organs has its own season. What does this mean? This means that if you have a predisposition for a weakness in an organ the problem will most likely come up during its own season. Organs work harder in their own season. More people suffer from heart attacks in the summer than at any other time of the year. Asthma, a condition of the lungs, is more prevalent in the autumn. When the seasons change pay attention to your stomach and spleen.

When you have this knowledge you can save yourself a lot of hassle and expense by strengthening your body *before* the beginning of each new season. Don't forget that *prevention is the highest medicine.* You can prevent the worsening of a chronic condition and stop problems developing from weak organs by beginning treatment a month *before* the season associated with that organ.

For example, if you suffer from respiratory problems (such as asthma, bronchitis, pneumonia or emphysema), they probably will flair up in autumn. Therefore, head them off at the pass strengthening your lungs at the end of summer to before autumn, lung season, begins. If you suffer from kidney ailments, sciatica or lumbago, begin treatment in autumn (before the cold days begin) to prevent a flair up in winter.

What type of treatment would be appropriate? A healthy diet is the first thing to consider. (That's why Chapter One was all about food.) Then there are herbs that are great to support the various organs.

Let's get back to Yin and Yang. Remember our friends from Chapter 1?

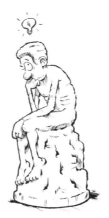

Here is a Yin position

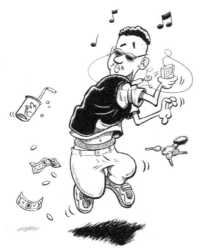

Here is a Yang position

Now, take a look at yourself. If you generally sit with your arms and legs crossed, if you often feel cold, if you are very thin, if you don't talk too much or if you don't have to run to the bathroom very often then your body is more Yin and you are more likely to develop a Yin (cold) ailment in moments of weakness.

All stiffness in the body is Yin. For example, colds, chilly fingers and toes, muscle and joint stiffness and depression are all signs of too much Yin in your body.

If you are very active, speak loudly, perspire a lot, feel hot, sit with your arms and legs apart, are quick to react and emotional, then your body has more Yang and you will be more likely to develop a Yang (hot) ailment.

All excess heat in the body is Yang. For example, fever, excess perspiration, thirst, nervousness and constipation are signs that there's too much Yang in your body.

Of course, this isn't black and white. These examples are extreme cases and people change according to circumstance. However, take it as a guideline and follow me.

Look out of the window. What kind of a day is it out there? When the weather is humid the body becomes "sticky". All the water in the body is "sticky" not liquid; more like oil. Travelling to a humid climate and not adjusting your food accordingly results in lethargy and heaviness. The body needs some stimulation to achieve better balance.

When the weather is hot and humid drink Yin tea, eat fresh fruit and salad to ease the flow of liquid in your body. Heavy foods like meat and rich foods like dairy products create a "stickiness" in your body. It is important not to use too much salt or sugar. These are two extreme substances and will create an "internal steam bath" by collecting water, which the body cannot control. The water will be retained in the body resulting in swollen legs and a bloated, heavy feeling. Eat light foods and drink lots of spring water.

If the day is cold and rainy enjoy a hearty stew or bake up a batch of delicious gingersnaps. You'll find a recipe at the end of the book.

Coffee and Tea

I'm not going to tell you "Never drink coffee". I can hear the sighs of relief. I do want you to be aware of *when* you drink it and what exactly happens when you do.

Coffee is Yin but it has a Yang manifestation in your body. How's that for a twist? A cup of coffee stimulates your body by creating little spasms in your small blood vessels that raise your blood pressure and wake you up.

Hot English tea (black tea) works the same way. It's good to drink it in places that have a cold, damp climate; just like England. Well, fancy that.

Green tea (Chinese tea) is Yin. It calms the body and is good to drink in hot, humid climates; such as Southern China.

Tannin in tea and caffeine in coffee are *drugs*. All drugs, of overused, can cause the body to shake. Sometimes the body needs a little stimulation, but remember that these substances are strong and use them consciously.

Now is a good time to mention "demon alcohol". If you drink alcohol, which is Yin, in moderation it can be useful to stimulate Yin organs such as the pancreas and liver to produce digestive juices, which help to digest food. If you slip from moderate use into excess use, alcohol will damage those organs.

Any chronic excess of either Yin or Yang damages your system.

Food controls the balance, which is precisely why it is so important to know how to use it. You can choose the food you eat much more easily than you can control the weather.

Now let's look at another cycle - Day and night. Guess what time is the most Yang?

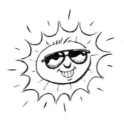

That's right. Noon is the most Yang time of day. The sun is at its strongest. After noon the sun has passed its highest point and the day progresses towards night. Midnight is the most Yin time, when all the world is quiet and dark.

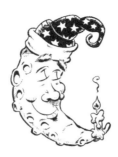

It's useful to know that the Chinese associate different times of day with the different organs of the body; at two-hour intervals different organs are at their peak energy level.

Here is a chart that shows which organs are associated with the hours of the day. The day is divided into twelve two-hour parts. Each part has one organ. Knowing which is which is very helpful in finding out the root cause of a problem. I'll explain more about how this works later. For now, have a look at the chart.

Time	Organ	Association
5 A.M. - 7 A.M.	Large Intestine	If you need to use the restroom now, it's a sign of good health
7 A.M. - 9 A.M.	Stomach	Eat breakfast
9 A.M. - 11 A.M.	Spleen	Digest your breakfast
11 A.M. - 1 P.M.	Heart	Coffee time
3 P.M. - 5 P.M.	Urine Bladder	Liquid out
5 P.M. - 7 P.M.	Kidney	Tea Time (Liquid in)
7 P.M. - 9 P.M.	Pericardium	Light meal
11 P.M. - 1 A.M.	Gall Bladder	Nighty-night
1 A.M. - 3 A.M.	Liver	Your body is rebuilding now
3 A.M. - 5 A.M.	Lungs	Sweet dreams

Is there a certain time of the day when your energy seems lower? At what time do you have the most energy? Do you regularly wake up at a particular time during the night? Do you usually go to the bathroom in the morning or later in the day? After evaluating some of these things, refer to the chart above and also the illustration below, which can give you a better understanding of the relationship between the time of day and specific organ function.

If, for instance, you are waking up at a certain time every night, make a note of the time, find it on the chart and notice the organ that is associated with that time. You may have a little weakness in that organ. Great. Now that you know about it you can support that organ so it doesn't have to get really sick for you to *do something* for it.

"What do I do?" you ask.

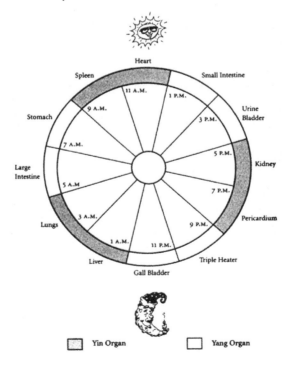

First of all *observe* yourself. Get used to paying attention to what is going on in your body at different times of the day. For example, look at 5-7 am on the chart above. That is the time of the Large Intestine. In other words, it's more or less the correct time to go to the toilet and empty the recycling bin. If you are in a state of good health then you are probably, naturally and easily eliminating your personal waste products daily at this time.

If you suffer from constipation it is a sign that your intestines are dry. Dryness is a Yang condition so you need more Yin food like fresh fruits and vegetables because they will create moisture in your system. Are you beginning to see how this works?

If you have the opposite condition and suffer from diarrhea it is a sign that you have an excess of dampness, an extreme Yin condition, in your intestines - wet, wet, wet. You need to gradually increase the Yang energy by drinking a cup of strong black tea (no sugar) and boiling up a hot stew of carrots and rice.

If you need a clothespin to put on your nose or you have to leave the bathroom window wide open maybe you should give a thought to your digestion: Strong odor comes from undigested foods, especially animal proteins. Be aware that the process of digestion starts in your mouth. Eat slowly and chew your food well so that you get a head start on digestion. There's more about the digestive process in the next chapter.

5 A.M. to 7 A.M. is Large Intestine Time. As mentioned before, this is the appropriate time to use the bathroom. If you are a healthy individual, you are more than likely eliminating waste products around this time naturally,

7 A.M. - 9 A.M. is Stomach Time. This is time for a nourishing breakfast. Don't skip this meal; it provides your fuel for the day. The food you eat at that time has the best chance of being completely digested. Maybe the Australians are on the right track with steak and eggs for breakfast.

9 A.M. -11 A.M. is Spleen Time. One of the spleen's functions is to support the stomach and finish off the digestive process that is started. I'll tell you more about the spleen in the next chapter.

11 A.M. – 1 P.M. is Heart Time. Bitter taste feeds the heart so if you want a cup of coffee this is a good time to have it. In England, work stops for "Elevenses". That's what they call their mid-morning coffee break.

1 P.M. - 3 P.M. is Small Intestine Time. In other words, a good time to eat lunch.

3 P.M. – 5 P.M. is Urine Bladder Time. Your bladder is most active at this time. It's getting pretty full and it's time to visit the bathroom and get rid of the liquid waste.

5 P.M. - 7 P.M. is Kidney Time. A cup of herbal tea increases the fluid in your body and will help to flush out your kidneys. It's also a good time for a catnap.

7 P.M. – 9 P.M. is Pericardium Time. The pericardium is the sack that surrounds and protects the heart. I'll tell you more about your pericardium in the next chapter. For now, it's enough to know that this is

the time to unwind, to calm down after your busy day, and a good time to cuddle with your partner.

9 P.M. - 11 P.M. is Triple Heater Time. It's best not to eat too much during this time – you don't want to burn your triple heater. It's what Western medicine called "the autonomic nervous system". It controls and balances all the other organs, supporting them with energy. This is the time when the body's automatic systems begin to work harder, processing the intake of the day and rebalancing your body by night.

11 P.M. – 1 A.M. is Gall Bladder Time. Have you ever had the experience of not being able to sleep after eating a particularly heavy dinner? This is your gall bladder running on overdrive; the hum of its motor keeps you awake.

1 A.M – 3 A.M is Liver Time. Your liver, the main factory in your body, is active at this time. If you often have disturbing dreams and wake up at this time, your liver probably needs some support.

3 A.M – 5 A.M is Lung Time. This is the time of deep, deep sleep. While you slumber, your lungs are working hard. Oxygen is the connection between the inside of your body and the outside environment. Most of the nutrients from the food you eat need oxygen to convert them into energy that your body can use. If you wake up at this time wheezing or have trouble breathing, there is probably a weakness of energy on your lungs.

This brings us back to 5 A.M. to 7 A.M. – Large Intestine Time – Good morning!

It is best not too eat too much in the evening. This is a time when the body's automatic systems begin to work harder, processing the intake of the day and rebalancing your body throughout the night. Notice the time that you wake up during the night, especially if it's every night. It may indicate a weakness in the organ that related to the time that your sleep is disturbed. For example, if you wake up around 3 A.M., your liver probably needs some support.

If you have any sort of infection (common symptoms of infections are a temperature, sore throat, runny nose, diarrhea, vaginal discharge) don't feed it sugar. Bacteria and viruses that cause infections thrive on sugar and sweets. If you want them to go away, starve them by taking away their favorite food.

Garlic is *great*. Use garlic during the cold and flu season to prevent infections. It is a natural antibiotic. Garlic also helps to lower high blood pressure by dissolving accumulated fat and cholesterol. It also stimulates digestion. Add one or two cloves of fresh garlic near the end of cooking. Overcooking garlic destroys some of its healthful properties.

Some helpful herbs and spices that you may already have in your kitchen:

Chamomile: A cup of chamomile tea is very good for digestive problems, insomnia, tension and menstrual cramps. It stabilizes and calms the energy of the stomach and intestines. If your tummy is upset in the morning (stomach hours) then drink chamomile tea. It's very good for soothing the discomfort of morning sickness. You can also use chamomile tea for eye irritations. Put some warm (not hot) tea on a piece of cotton and bathe your eyelids.

Mint: Mint tea is good to relax and cool the body. It promotes circulation of bile in the Liver and Gall Bladder and relieves discomfort in the upper right-hand side of the abdomen. It disperses accumulated energy there and can help relieve a migraine headache if the root of the headache is in the Liver and Gall Bladder (more on this subject later) If you feel uncomfortable late at night and in the early hours of the morning then try drinking a cup of mint tea. Mint tea works great to ease a hangover. Even better, if you can remember to take a cup of mint tea in between your drinks then you can avoid a hangover all together. (How I know this? I have to admit it's through personal experience.)

Cinnamon: This spice is *numero uno* (the best) for promoting circulation in the heart and supporting your kidneys. It warms the entire body, creating a kind of internal central heating system. You can use cinnamon sticks to brew up a pot of tea or add powdered cinnamon to coffee, cocoa or even food.

Licorice: Drinking Licorice tea cleanses and detoxifies the body. It stimulates both the spleen and stomach and supports the digestive system as well as strengthening the lungs. It is also very good for children who have a lack of appetite. By regularly drinking licorice tea toxins are eliminated before they can cause damage to the body. Licorice is a great preventative and curative medicine - and it tastes good, too.

Ginger: This spice warms the body and helps digestion. It also warms the stomach, spleen and intestines. If you have a weakness in your digestion system drink a cup of ginger tea half an hour after your main meal or between 7 A.M and 11 A.M, the times of your stomach and spleen.

Speaking of the spleen... who knows what the spleen does? Or what a gall bladder does besides making stones that shouldn't be there? For a simple introduction to the inner you - read on.

3 The Inside Story

In this chapter I will give you a little bit of information about what is going on inside you. It's time to meet the in-laws; those strange and unfamiliar beings that are a part of the family but not very familiar.

One cell from a woman and one cell from a man meet. They swim together in a beautiful dance of life. And what do they do?

Two cells join together to create a new motion of life.

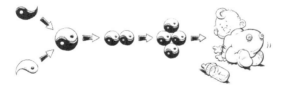

Through motion they expand their life force and divide and multiply - the two become four, the four become sixteen, the sixteen become 256 and so on and so on until after about three months there is a teeny, tiny *you* swimming around its mother's womb; a little fish with its mothers eyes and its father's nose.

This motion is called *Organogenisis* or for those who don't speak Greek - "The Birth of the Organs". By three months all the major organs have formed. They continue to grow and develop; each as a vital part of the whole, holy human. Let's take a look at some parts of the human body and the role these parts play in the whole that is *you*.

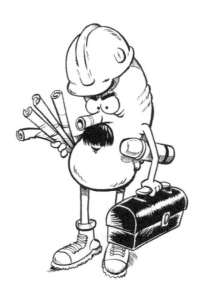

Kidneys

Your Kidneys are the "Boss". They hold the genetic blueprints that have the instructions on how everything else works. They are the main battery of the body - the power source that keep things going. One of the Boss's duties is to filter your blood. Your kidneys remove toxins from your blood and allow what remains to continue on around your body providing fuel for your cells. The toxins are eliminated in the form of urine, which is stored in your Urine Bladder until it's time to go...to the bathroom! Your kidneys control the function of your ears, bones, joints and reproductive organs.

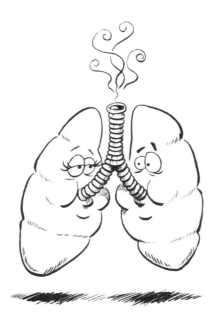

Lungs

Your Lungs are the processing plant for oxygen, one of your body's two main fuels. Our first and last connection with the outside world is through a *breath*. Oxygen in the air is processed by the lungs and sent to all your cells via your blood as it circulates through your body dropping off oxygen and collecting carbon dioxide. It returns to the lungs where the carbon dioxide is removed and leaves your body when you exhale. AAAHHHHH! Your lungs control the quality of your skin.

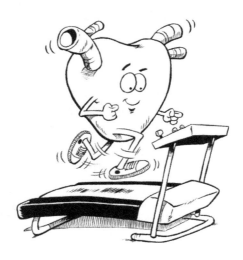

Heart

Your Heart pumps blood all throughout your body. Your blood carries oxygen in and carbon dioxide out and also regulates your body's temperature. It transports nutrients from the food you eat into your cells and carries waste products away. Oxygen and nutrients are the two fuels that keep your body running.

The Chinese say "Your spirit dwells in your heart." What does that mean? It means that the energy of your heart inspires your deepest thoughts and dreams. Love is the energy of your heart; your spirit. The energy of your heart is expressed verbally by what you say and how you say it. Free and relaxed communication makes you lighthearted and happy.

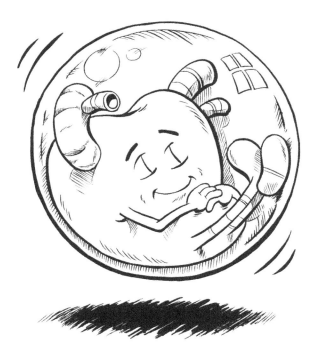

Pericardium

Your Pericardium (what's that?) is a kind of sack around your heart. I think of it as a nest that cuddles and protects your heart from emotional stress, helping it do its job of circulating your blood. It also influences your hormonal system.

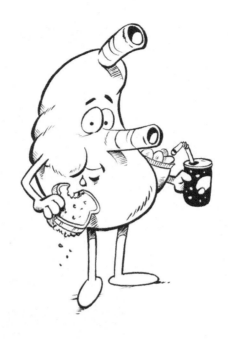

Stomach

Your Stomach breaks down proteins and prepares other food so it can be absorbed and enter your blood in a form that the body can use. The process of digestion starts in your mouth. When you chew your food well saliva is produced. The action of saliva on the food starts the digestive process. When lunch reaches your stomach the fluids there break down the proteins. The proteins, which are now broken up into little pieces and the rest of the food, which isn't (especially if you ate quickly and didn't chew it well) go into the Small Intestine.

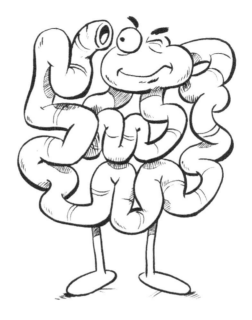

Small Intestine

Your Small Intestine, is where food is mainly absorbed. Close your eyes and picture a twenty-foot-long hose all coiled up in your belly. Imagine the tube lined with fur. Your blood flows into the tiny strands and picks up the nutrients that have been absorbed by the small intestine. Spy cells are on the lookout for fat. When they identify fat they get on their cell phones and call your Gall Bladder.

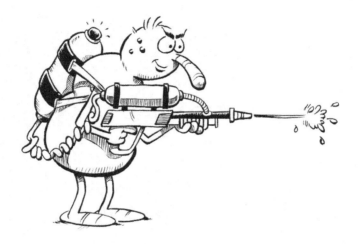

Gall Bladder

Your Gall Bladder sends a shot of bile into the small intestine. Bile is a digestive juice that breaks down fat so that it can be absorbed by the small intestine. (Imagine a turkey baster squirting out a shot of bile.) The proteins that were broken down in the stomach continue to be digested and are absorbed into the small intestine and from there flow into your bloodstream.

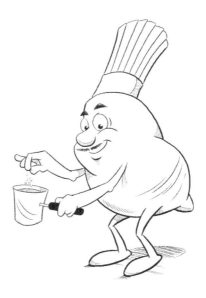

Liver

After absorbing nutrients in your small intestine, the enriched blood must pass through your liver, the body's main factory. This is where all the magic happens. Your digestive system breaks down the food you eat into its basic components. In your liver all these building blocks are reassembled into a kind of nuclear fuel. All the various types of fuel that the different parts of your body require are assembled in your liver – the master chef that turns raw ingredients onto your personal favorite dish. The whole smorgasbord is served up though your bloodstream, and each part of your body takes what it needs to energize and build it.

Your liver cleans your blood and recycles it. In addition, it stores extra blood that is not currently needed for circulation, acting rather like a Fort Knox for the body, providing essential reserves in case of massive blood loss through injury. Your liver produces the bile that is stored in the gall bladder; this bile is used to break down fat. And look! The state of your liver also has an effect on your eyes and your vision. Evaluating these two things is a good way to measure the condition of this organ.

Yet another way to assess the quality of your liver is to look at your nails. If they are strong and healthy, so is your liver.

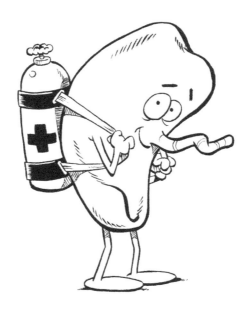

Spleen

Your Spleen is a storehouse for blood that may be needed in an emergency. In case of infection your spleen sends troops of white blood cells to the rescue. Your spleen is also the "old folks home" for blood. After traveling around your body for three or four months, red blood cells go to your spleen to relax and take it easy. When they die their parts are recycled by your Spleen into brand new blood. Your lips and mouth show the condition of your spleen.

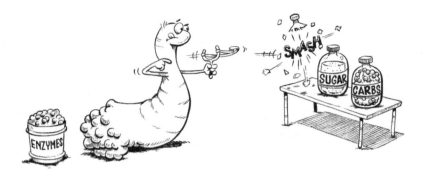

Pancreas

Partially digested sugar and carbohydrates in the small intestine activate your Pancreas, a fish shaped organ with two jobs. Its first job is to send out enzymes that break up sugar and carbohydrates into small pieces so they can be absorbed into the blood. The blood then carries the sugar to the cells and the cells use the sugar as fuel to give the body energy. Its second job is to produce the hormone insulin.

What does insulin do and why do we need it? Your blood is the transport that carries oxygen and nutrients from your food to all the cells in your body. Each cell is a complete unit that needs energy to live. Sugar provides the fuel that keeps the cell working, much like gas in a car. Fats and proteins build and support the function of each cell.

But how does that energy get inside? Digested proteins and fat enter cells easily. They have a key to the front door. But poor old sugar doesn't have a key. It needs a doorkeeper to let it in. This is what insulin is - it is the doorkeeper that allows sugar to enter a cell. If a cell does not have sugar to burn as fuel then it will burn fat instead. That's why eliminating sugar from your diet will help you lose the fat that your body has stored for a rainy day. If you have no more fat to burn, then the hungry cells will look for another source of fuel. It is at this point that they start to use the protein inside of themselves, which is very harmful to your body.

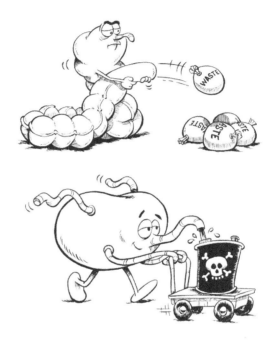

Large Intestine & Urine Bladder

Your Large Intestine and Urine Bladder prepare and store solid and liquid waste for recycling - outside of your body.

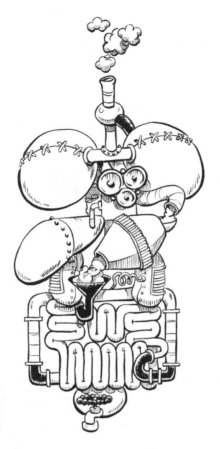

Triple Heater

Your Triple Heater (never heard of it?) is not a physical organ. This one is a little tricky to explain. Remember the story of the teapot that I told you in the introduction to this book? The triple heater I a good example of that story – different cultures observe the same thing from different viewpoints and then draw different conclusions. In Chinese medicine, harmony between the different organs is considered even more important than the health of each organ individually. The first phase of treatment is to harmonize the entire body and then to focus on the effected organ. In contrast, Western medicine concentrates on curing (or removing!) the diseased organ.

So here's how the triple heater works: Imagine your trunk being divided into three sections. In the top section are your lungs and your heart. Breathing and purification of your blood happens here. In the middle section, digestion takes place in your stomach, liver, spleen and pancreas. The lower part, below your navel, is where your kidneys, intestines and reproductive organs are housed. This is the main recycling center where the useful is separated from the useless and your personal waste is eliminated. The triple heater coordinates the functions of these three sections so that they all work together in harmony. It controls the temperature of the water in your cells, keeping everything at body temperature, the ideal level of warmth to keep everything running smoothly.

From the Western point of view, the triple heater's job is done by your hormones and your autonomic nervous system – that is, all the things that keep on working without your having to do anything about it. Hormones are produced in your glands. If your body is a factory, then the glands are the managers. The general manager is your pituitary gland, situated right between your eyes, nestled within your brain. It is responsible for all the other glands, like the thyroid, adrenal glands, gonads, etc. As your blood flows through the glands, it picks up instructions in the form of hormones. Hormones trigger specific organs into action. They are very potent; a little goes a long way. To know what is needed where, the general manager uses the world's most remarkable super-computer - your brain.

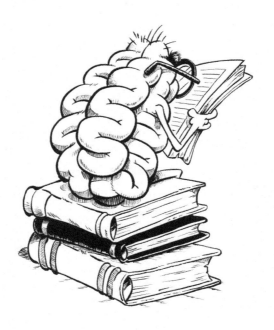

Brain

Your brain is the center of consciousness, thought, intellect and memory. It controls the functions of seeing, hearing, smelling and speaking. The rich capillary system in your brain circulates a large amount of blood that provides a way of receiving information about the other organs. Another communication system is the spinal marrow and nerves - your personal information super-highway.

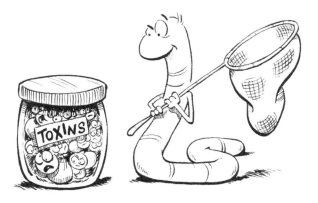

Appendix

Your appendix looks like a little worm and about as long as your index finger. Although it's "appended" to your intestines, it is part of the body's defense system along with your tonsils and lymph nodes. Your appendix and tonsils are made of the same type of tissue and produce "defender" cells that seek, capture and eliminate bacteria, viruses and toxins, vagrants who have no place in a healthy body. Your tonsils are the first line of defense. They catch what they can before the enemy gets very far into your body. Your appendix catches toxins during digestion. Your spleen sends out cells that attack any bacteria, toxins or viruses that manage to enter your bloodstream. The heat of this battle causes your temperature to rise.

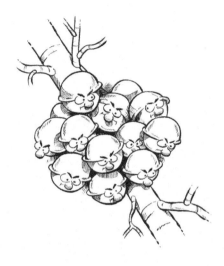

Lymph Nodes

Your lymph nodes look like small bunches of grapes and are located around all your major organs and blood vessels. They provide a base for white blood cells to hang out until they are needed. The lymph nodes are involved in the first line of defense to stop the spread of infection in your body. If you cut your finger, the very first thing to react is your blood. White blood cells rush to the scene of the accident to fight off and kill bacteria. If they are not strong enough to do it alone or if the cut is very large and overwhelming, then the white cells e-mail a message to the lymph nodes under your arms to send re-enforcements, ASAP.

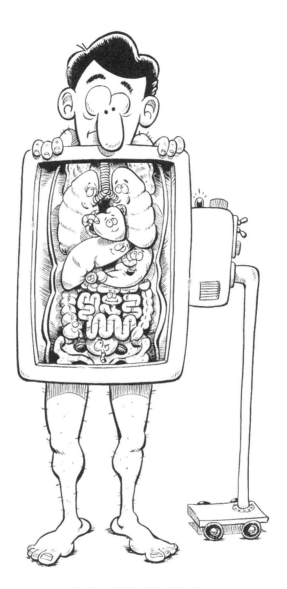

The Whole Body

You can see how interdependent all these systems are. A weakness in one of them will cause a weakness in all the others. Of course, there is a lot more going on in your body than this, but I wanted to give you a simple overview of what your friends inside of you are busy doing, twenty-four hours a day, every day of your life. Take a look at the full body diagram above: notice how the organs fit snugly together – each is so very dependent upon the others. Because of this interconnectedness, all of the organs must be in harmony, with themselves and with each other, for an overall healthy and smooth running system.

A Look at Some Common Imbalances

First, I'd like to talk about diabetes. Diabetes is a condition that occurs when the pancreas cannot produce enough insulin to allow sugar to be absorbed into the cells. Some people have a genetic predisposition to develop diabetes. If these people don't pay attention to what they eat there is a good chance that they will develop the disease. This is what happens: if a person with a genetic predisposition to diabetes eats sugar, sweet foods or overindulges in alcohol every day, then over the years, the insulin producing cells in the pancreas that are already weak burn out and die from being overworked. When less insulin is produced sugar cannot be absorbed into the cells and used for fuel. The sugar stays in the blood (you've probably heard of "high blood sugar"). Too much sugar in the blood corrodes the capillaries and, after a while, they become rigid and unable to do their job of absorbing nutrients and oxygen. Generally, after ten to fifteen years, people with unchecked diabetes will begin to have problems with their eyes, kidneys and joints. These places have rich capillary systems that become damaged over time by too much sugar in the blood that flows through them.

People who have a family history of diabetes need to pay attention to the way they live. It is important that they avoid eating sugar or sweets and that they work in low-stress jobs. The onset of diabetes is preventable. If you feel thirsty all the time, have a dryness in your mouth, feel nervous, if you get "the shakes" and craving for sugar then you had better get the situation checked out. Sugar cravings are caused when cells are hungry for sugar. There could be plenty in your blood but without insulin to unlock the door to the cell they "hear it knocking - but it can't get in." If the condition has already developed, then medication is needed. In addition to the prescribed medication, eating the correct food and drinking a mixture of ginger, celery and parsley juice everyday will help to counteract the high level of sugar in the blood.

Now let's talk about another ailment. I'm sure you've heard of gallstones, but do you know what they are or what causes them? If there are bacteria in the gall bladder they can cause an infection that changes the quality of the bile. It gets sticky and acts like glue, sticking to the bacteria and dead cells. More and more of it accumulates and sticks. Eventually, like a pearl, many layers build up and create a "stone". These vary in quantity, shape and size. They can be as tiny as a grain of sand or as large as a marble. The gall bladder is like a neat little pear shaped sack. The stones irritate its inside walls. They are sometimes pulled out of the gall bladder into the small intestine along with the normal bile flow and are eliminated. That's the good news. The bad news is that sometimes they get stuck in the bile duct (the little tube that connects the gall bladder to the small intestine). If this happens the flow of bile is blocked. This leads to problems with digestion and causes a bile build-up in the gall bladder and liver, which makes the skin and the whites of the eyes take on a yellowish coloring and can cause a sharp pain just under the ribs on the right-hand side; in other words: big trouble!

If you have your gall bladder removed, your liver kindly takes over the job of sending bile into your intestine to let you digest fat. However, unlike the gall bladder, which squirts out a blast of bile when you need it most, the liver just lets it drip continuously, whether you need it or not. So, if you don't have a gall bladder, don't eat too much fat at once.

It's Your Choice

Let's talk briefly about smoking. What about it? If you don't smoke, don't start. If you already smoke, one cigarette after lunch will not kill you. Nicotine stimulates your digestive juices but if you smoke too much, or smoke without eating, you will damage your stomach and lungs. Smoking will, in fact, damage all your systems because it creates an imbalance in your internal central heating system. So, if you cannot restrict yourself to one cigarette after meals it is better to quit - *soon*. If you do enjoy that after-dinner cigarette, be aware that other people around you who don't smoke might not want to share it with you. Make a point never to smoke around babies or small children.

Now, let's move on to soft drinks. An often over-looked source of trouble in the West is the widespread consumption of carbonated drinks. We won't mention any names. Besides the fact that most carbonated drinks contain a huge amount of sugar (or equally unhealthy sugar substitute) the carbonation in the drink masquerades as digestive juice (and this includes carbonated water) This makes the real digestive juice producers in your body lazy. Your digestive system becomes dependent on carbonated drinks to do its job. It's all right to have a carbonated drink occasionally or when you need to bring up a burp -- but *not* every day

4 A Tale of Two Headaches

Mary has a headache. Jane has a headache, too. They can both take two aspirins and call me in the morning. Maybe they'll feel better for a while, but the chances are that they will both call me back again next week complaining of another headache. Why?

Most headache medicines on the market may be effective pain relievers, but they do not address the *cause* of the headache. Until you identify and treat the cause, the problem will keep coming back to haunt you. Always remember, *not all headaches are created equal.*

First I'll tell you about Mary. Mary is in her forties. She's been having headaches a couple of times a week for the last few months. When the headache begins, she gets very sensitive to noise and to light. She likes to be alone in a darkened room until the pain subsides. She experiences a sharp pain that stretches from one eyebrow to the top of her ear on one side of her head. This kind of headache is commonly known as a migraine.

Mary is unhappy with her job. She is rather short-tempered and often has cravings for chocolate. From my experience, her symptoms indicate that the root of her headache is a problem with her digestion. This stems from an imbalance between her Liver and Gall Bladder caused by continuous stress in her lifestyle and by eating the wrong foods.

What would I recommend to Mary? First of all, I would suggest that she change her diet. Nix the coffee, alcohol and hot spices. Forget about chocolate and sweets. When Mary craves chocolate she can make herself a morning cup of hot cocoa. (Mix one teaspoon of <u>unsweetened</u> cocoa powder and one teaspoon of honey into a quarter cup of hot milk.

When the cocoa has dissolved add more hot milk to fill the cup. Cocoa is rich in iron that supports the blood but has none of the sugar and fat of processed chocolate.) Mary needs to eat more salads, green vegetables and fresh fruit to harmonize her stomach and to take in more minerals to strengthen her blood. Soups, salad, fresh dandelion greens and fruit will calm her body and support the flow of energy in her liver. She would benefit from a cup of mint tea in the afternoon and before she goes to bed at night.

It would also be a good idea to find a job that she enjoys doing. Anger and frustration at spending time at a job you hate slowly builds up and poisons your liver.

Now let's meet Jane. Jane is in her sixties, retired and has a calm disposition. When she gets a headache, she feels pain in the back of her head. It's worse when the weather starts to get cold. She often has aches and stiffness in her neck, her shoulders and sometimes feels a dull pain in her lower back. Jane complains of eyestrain when her headaches begin. She has an accumulation of cold in her body, a degenerative process (osteoporosis) in her vertebrae and weak blood circulation in her upper back and neck. It is the weak circulation and accumulated cold that causes her headaches. Her problem is worse when the thermometer drops.

Jane needs hot drinks, especially cinnamon or ginger tea to aid her digestion, promote the circulation of her blood and warm up all her body. She should eliminate cold foods like ice cream and iced drinks. She should avoid any extreme foods (see the seesaws in chapter 1) Rice and soup with a little spice added to them will warm her up. Jane should invest in a warm scarf and make sure that her neck and back are kept toasty. A magnetic belt would do her a lot of good and a sauna would be beneficial to really warm up her toes. Light exercise, slow head rolls, stretching, yoga and anything that develops flexibility in her back and neck will help Jane to avoid headaches in the future.

Here are a few more examples of common headaches and where their origins. Mike is a teenager. He's tall and gangly, 16 years old, just got his driver's license and can't wait to get on with his life. Like many teenagers he's nervous, tense and temperamental. His eating habits are bad: he prefers to hang out with his friends and grab some grub at the mall, he eats too quickly and washes down his food with lots of ice cold cola rather than staying at home for a leisurely home-cooked meal. Lately, headaches and stomach aches have been cramping his style; not only that, but he has to burp all the time and sometimes even vomits..

Mike's headaches and upset stomach usually hit right after he eats. Their source is Mike's weak stomach, which is due to poor eating habits- both in style and content. First of all, Mike needs to *eat slowly*. He needs to eliminate cola, spicy food, fried foods and, for the time being, meat. "Oh man!" I hear him say. "What *can* I eat?" If Mike wants to eat at home he can have lots of good food. He can start his day with a cup of licorice tea. For lunch and dinner, soup is great, accompanied by boiled foods, vegetables, yogurt and fresh fruit. But, if Mike just can't break away from the gang he can still find things to eat that will be better than what he was eating before. Many fast food places offer soup or salad – both are good choices. He can find a place that serves pasta with a non-spicy sauce or eat vegetarian Chinese food. But he *cannot* drink cola.

I have already mentioned that carbonated drinks weaken the digestive system. In fact, drinking any liquid with food is not a good idea. Only "civilized" human beings drink water with their meals. Animals know to eat first and then drink. Maybe we can learn something from them. Drinking liquids with meals will dilute your digestive juices. You know what that means.

The main thing for Mike and for all of us to remember is to pay more attention to the food we eat - not just the kind of food but also how we eat it. When we read the paper or watch television while we eat, our brain disconnects from our stomach. Good digestion starts before we even begin to eat: We may see a delicious looking meal on television or smell good food cooking. These things produce saliva in our mouths, readying them for the intake of a meal. If you don't pay attention to the food you are eating or if you eat food that is unappetizing then your body produces less digestive juice and you can develop a "lazy stomach" leading to problems with your digestion. *fast food = fast death*.

Mike needs to watch his diet very carefully for a couple weeks. After that, yogurt and cereal will start his day off well. Fresh fruit in his pocket and fresh vegetables for lunch will keep him on the right track. He can start to eat meat again and have the *occasional* junk food meal and cola. But if he reverts to his previous way of eating, his headaches will return.

Meet Mike's Auntie Agnes. Agnes feels a dull pain all over her head. She's thirty years old and works as a secretary. Mike says, "Auntie Agnes always moves in slow motion." He thinks it's funny. Agnes doesn't. She's overweight, has a pale complexion, feels tired all the time and has no energy. She doesn't like to walk, to move or to do anything physical. She gets up in the morning and goes through her day like a zombie. She has no hopes or dreams and is not in a relationship. Every day she takes the bus to work. She always feels a dull ache in her head that gets worse in the afternoon. She often falls asleep in the bus on her way home and wakes up feeling worse. Poor Agnes. She's a mess!

Agnes's headache is caused by a lack of life force. The dull pain in her head comes from dullness in her whole body. She needs to recharge her blood and increase the circulation of blood in her body. To put it in the poetic terms of Chinese imagery: the energy in her body has pooled into a stagnant lake rather than a flowing river.

Agnes needs to shake herself by the shoulders and make some changes in her lifestyle. The first thing that she needs to do is *move*. Instead of taking the bus all the way to work she can get off one block earlier and walk the rest of the way. In the evening she can do the same thing on her way home. When that becomes comfortable then she can get off two blocks earlier.

At work she can nibble on beneficial snacks like strawberries, raspberries, blackberries rather eating candy or potato chips. Instead of coffee she can have fresh orange or carrot juice. A cup of stimulating cinnamon or ginger tea in the morning and mint tea in the afternoon and evening will help balance Agnes' system. Agnes must forget about junk food, caffeine, nicotine, chocolate and sodas. When she starts to feel more alive, she can find something she likes to do that will provide both exercise and social contact, such as taking a dance class or playing softball every weekend.

Let's meet one more lady. Her name is Sally. She doesn't get headaches very often. Usually she feels pretty good. She leads an active life, eats well, and has a well-paying job that she loves. She's happily married with two lovely children and she finds time to go to aerobic classes twice a week. She's a Super Mom, and has everything "under control." Today, though, Sally has a headache. She noticed that when she get a headache it's often just before her menstrual period starts. The pain throbs in her temples. This kind of headache is like a little wake up call. It says "Hey! Slow down and take care of your body!" What Sally needs is *rest*. It's time to tell the family, "Excuse me but I need to take care of *myself* now." A hot bath with a few drops of lavender oil, relaxing music, and a cup of mint, chamomile or valerian tea will calm her body, relax her muscles and regulate her sleep. Sally needs to put on the breaks. Her body needs time to renew and refresh itself.

It used to be that a woman would take to her couch when she had her menstrual period; it's a time that nature sets aside for women to refresh and renew their energy. These days, women don't have the luxury of quietly staying home during menstruation. Women, if you are aware that nature requires a little quiet time then make a gesture to accommodate it. Make a date with yourself to spend at least one quiet evening at home each month. Ask the family's indulgence. Don't answer the phone. Don't bring work home. For one night a month, just pamper yourself. Think of it as an investment in health.

Getting back to our headaches: Did you know that 80 percent of headaches are symptoms of a functional imbalance either between organs or between the body and its environment? When you are suffering from a headache, by all means take an aspirin or other mild painkiller. But when the pain subsides don't just sit there and wait for the next attack. Fight back! Start to make changes in your lifestyle and diet. If you smoke, quit. Walk, or start an exercise program. Tall orders, I know, but your life is at stake. Acupuncture can help a lot to ease the discomfort of transition to a healthier lifestyle. It tunes your body and helps to support the weaknesses that make changing difficult. I'll tell you more about how acupuncture works in Chapter 8.

If headaches still persist even after you have improved your life style, it is time to have a checkup to see if there is a localized, specific problem of the sinus, ears, eyes, nose, or teeth, genetic damage of blood vessels, a tumor or something else. If you have already made changes toward a healthier lifestyle your body will be in a much stronger position to tackle a more serious problem if that proves to be the cause of your pain.

5 Show Some Emotion

Someone said, "We are what we eat" but that's not enough. Descartes said, "I think therefore I am" but that is not complete. The philosopher John Donne said, "No man is an island." Now that's getting closer. We are all part of a greater whole. We experience our environment through our *feelings*; through the feeling of our five senses: sight, hearing, taste, touch and smell; through the feelings perceived as emotions; and through hunches and insights which are a sort of mental feeling.

All contact with our environment has an influence on our health. Without our five senses we would have no knowledge of the world around us. They allow us to interact with our environment. They allow us to survive and enjoy life. Our hunches and instincts also help us to survive, if we pay attention to them. People who live close to nature have more sensitive senses and keener perception. They are aware of the subtle changes of temperature and of the behavior of birds and animals. They have to be. Their survival depends on it.

As we became more technologically advanced, we learned to control our immediate environment. We live in comfortable houses with heating and cooling systems. Our food comes from the grocery store, rather than from hunting and gathering. All of this gives us more time for other things, like developing arts and technology or watching TV.

However, our survival still depends on our interaction with the world through the food we eat, the air we breathe and the relationships we form. As well as getting information about our physical environment we also get information about the other people who share it with us. This brings me to the next piece of the puzzle of total health: *emotions*!

Do you know the difference between a feeling and an emotion? A feeling is what you actually experience. Feelings show in your body. For example, if you get angry you face might flush, your fists might clench; you might feel tension in your jaw. You know you're angry. The emotion that goes with that feeling is more complicated: it involves a judgment about that feeling; a judgment usually based on past experiences of feeling angry. Your reactions to the emotion of anger can be very disproportional to the situation at hand the event that produced the feeling of anger. It's important to observe how you react when faced with a strong feeling or emotion. In order to stay healthy, it's good to learn the trick of acknowledging your feelings without getting carried away by the emotion. It takes some practice, to be sure, but the first step is realizing the difference.

You can think of feelings as the strings of a guitar and emotions as the sound that comes out when they are strummed. The sound depends on how tight the strings are. If they are too tight then the sound is hard. If they are too loose then the sound is weak. The trick is to have the strings at just the right tension and tuned in relationship to one another so that the resulting sound is harmonious.

As you can see from this example, feelings and emotions take on physical form in your body. Continuous strong emotions directly affect the different organs in your body. Here is the chart that shows some of the correspondences (Chinese style) between organs, emotions and other interesting things that you might not have considered were related to one another.

Yin Organ	Liver	Heart	Lungs	Kidney	Spleen
Yang Organ	Gall Bladder	Small Intestine	Large Intestine	Urine Bladder	Stomach
Facial Feature	Eyes	Tongue	Nose	Ears	Lips
Season	Spring	Summer	Autumn	Winter	The end of each season
Emotion	Anger	Happiness Unhappiness	Sadness	Fear	Nervous-ness Worry
Body Connection	Ligaments/ Tendons	Blood Vessels	Skin	Bones/ Bone marrow	Muscles
Energy	Wind	Heat	Dryness	Coldness	Dampness
Taste	Sour	Bitter	Pungent	Salty	Sweet
Element	Wood	Fire	Metal	Water	Earth

Sadness affects your lungs. Think of all those nineteenth century stories in which the star-crossed lover expires from tuberculosis. Lungs are paired with the large intestines. Sadness can cause a blockage of energy in them, a sluggishness that leads to constipation. If sadness is a part of your life take a walk in nature, breathe deeply, listen to the birds singing and know that the sadness will pass.

Anger affects your liver and gall bladder. In my language we have the expression, "I was so angry I vomited bile". In English, you say, "I was so angry I saw red." The eyes, you remember, are associated with the liver.

When you are feeling angry, stop and take a breath. Observe where you are holding the anger in your body; in your fists? In your jaw? Consciously relax your body when you exhale. If you have a buildup of unexpressed anger, find a place where you can *yell*. Go to a local sporting event or to a noisy highway and yell until you feel the anger releasing. Singing is another good way to relieve unexpressed anger. Join a choir. Let go with a scream or a song while you're driving (if you don't have a convertible, that is); just remember to keep your eyes open.

Joy! What's wrong with that? How can we have too much joy? Well, let's say you've just heard about the birth of your first grandchild or that you won $64 million in the lottery. A pleasant shock, but a shock nonetheless. If your heart is weak you may spend all your winnings on doctor's bills. Too much of a good thing can weaken your heart and your small intestines. What to do? Relax and *exhale*! Joy is wonderful, but sometimes if you laugh too much it's hard to catch your breath. So remember to exhale.

Nervousness and worry affect your spleen and stomach. This is a very common condition in modern life. You worry about survival and about how to make ends meet. You get nervous in traffic; you have stress in your daily life. All of this creates an imbalance in your stomach. This imbalance sometimes causes over eating, cravings for the wrong food or a lack of appetite. You can be caught in a downward spiral of stomach problems. What to do? Change your habits or your job, if you can. Find work you enjoy and a mode of transportation that doesn't cause stress. Avoid eating hot or spicy foods and smoking. Make a point to eat at regular times and don't eat heavy food late in the evening. Make time to spend with your friends. Learn and practice anti-stress techniques such as deep breathing, meditation or yoga. *Relax, man.*

Fear. This is a big one. An infant who is startled will wet its pants. This is a natural reaction because fear directly affects the kidney and urine bladder. Adults learn to control and suppress this natural reaction. Thank goodness. But we don't learn what we can do to prevent a buildup of fear in our bodies. Fear is the deepest held emotion. It is the strongest and the most subtle. The "fight or flight" response is programmed into us. In today's society we must curb our natural instincts; feelings of fear get stuck and are held in our bodies.

The best we can do is to become *aware* of the fear that we are holding. It runs deep in our subconscious. Think of insurance. The whole concept is based on our fear that something awful is going to happen and we must somehow be "covered". When we watch the news, we see all the worst that society and nature have to offer. Good news is not news. Think about it. We are treated to stories of murder, theft, corruption, rape, accidents and natural disasters. All of this "news" makes us fearful that something like that can happen to us. Our brains switch off for a moment and we forget that the chances of something like that happening to us are, in reality, pretty slim. We need to keep a sense of perspective and rational thinking while being bombarded with all this negative information.

I'm not suggesting you live recklessly or take unnecessary chances but *don't let fear paralyze you*. Much of it is all in our imagination. Learn to moderate fear. Turn off the television or limit your viewing to programs on animals and see how they cope with life in the wild. Getting on top of fear is all about awareness. Respect the difficulties in your life and accept them, but see them for what they are, not blown out of all proportion into what they may become.

Remember, you don't experience one emotion at a time. Generally, you are presented with a lovely bouquet of emotions. Sometimes it's hard to realize exactly what is that you are feeling. That's when it's good to have a look at what's going on in your body for *clues*.

Emotions can lead to serious mental and physical problems if they are extreme and continuous and allowed to build up over time. Find moderation in your emotions. If your way of life is amiss you will find yourself in extreme situations that will eventually manifest in your physical body and destroy your health.

Spend more time doing what you like to do, doing things that make you happy. If you can't change your job right away, then make time for a hobby that you enjoy. Spend time with people you like and who share your interests. Being healthy includes having good company, pleasant times and humor.

Imagine you have an emotion quota. Any emotion can fill it up. So, why not fill it with happiness and pleasure? You'll find that there is less room for sadness, anger and fear. It's your choice, you know. In the immortal words of Bobbie McFerrin, *"Don't worry, be happy"*.

6 What You Can't See Can Hurt You

Now that you understand about Yin and Yang and have had a look at what's going on inside you, I'd like to spend some time explaining what is going on outside you, energetically, that can affect your health. And that is *plenty*.

One hundred years ago a television set would have been unimaginable. Now we take it for granted that someone miles away can be seen right there on our television screen. How about the magic of the remote control? Click, click and something happens to the television, apparently all by itself. Cellular phones extend the reach of your voice without any cords or wires. I think we all know that this "magic" is actually a physical phenomenon (something we learned about in physics class but have now totally forgotten.) The point is, we can't see anything but we know something is there.

It's common knowledge that there are a lot of stray waves flying through the air all the time that are produced by broadcast television, radio, microwaves, computers, cell phones, radar and powerful emissions from high-tension wires and high voltage power stations, for example.

These waves vibrate over a wide spectrum of frequencies. How do all the different waves affect us? Extensive research is being conducted in Europe, Japan and the United States to find out. Over the last few decades, as more and more technical equipment is being developed and widely used, there is a growing concern about their health consequences. People know from experience that exposure to these waves weakens their system. Now it's up to the scientists to explain why.

Less well known are the subtle vibrations that are under our feet; some are manmade and others occur naturally.

Our earth is a giant magnet. Its rotation produces electrical currents in the earth's molten metal core. These electro-magnetic currents create subtle, invisible vibrations that are everywhere - in the earth itself, in the air, in us and in every living thing. Life on earth evolved in accordance with these subtle but ever-present vibrations. All life is dependent on them to regulate the subtle vibrations within.

Imagine a grid of energetic "walls" about 8 inches wide that run north to south and east to west all around the globe.

The REAL World -wide-web

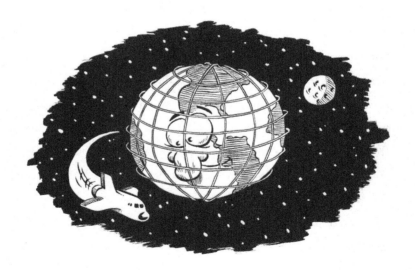

The ones running north to south are about six feet apart. The ones that run east to west are a little closer together. You can find these walls everywhere.

They can be disturbing to humans. If you spend a lot of time exposed to them, you may *feel tense, tired or weak*. Cats, on the other hand, really enjoy the energy that comes from these places. They seem to feel a comfortable warmth in there. Strange but true. So, don't sleep where your cat sleeps.

If the walls are uncomfortable then the spots where they cross are a pain. This is how they work:

Each line has a charge, either positive or negative. Where positive and negatively charged lines crossed the effect is minimal. However, on the spots where there is a double charge, either positive or negative, there's a double whammy.

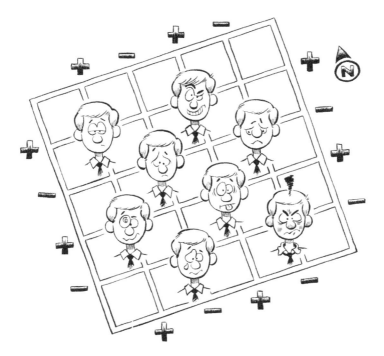

These hot spots are known in the trade as Hartmann Knots, after Dr. Ernst Hartmann who made this discovery. Here is an example of what a Hartmann Knot can do:

Mr. and Mrs. Smith are a young couple who used to be happily married, but lately there's been trouble in paradise. Mrs. Smith wakes up feeling tired every morning. She tosses and turns all night and all that movement bothers Mr. Smith. To top it all off, the light has gone out of their love life. Everything was fine until they moved into their new house a few months ago, but things have been going slowly downhill since then. Why? Let's have a look at the invisible walls in the Smiths' new bedroom and see what's happening.

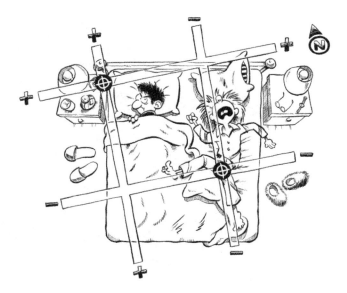

Mrs. Smith sleeps on an energetic wall. There is no way that she can have a good night's sleep there. She twists and turns all night, disturbing Mr. Smith. Have a look where the other line is. No wonder they never feel "in the mood" anymore. Every morning Mrs. Smith hits the snooze button, one, two, three times. When she finally crawls out of bed, she needs two cups of coffee just to open her eyes. If she continues to sleep in this place the chances are that she will develop a problem in her abdomen, womb or lower back because two walls cross right at that spot. The good news for this couple is that they can move their bed to a place that is not influenced by energetic walls. They will probably feel like popping open a bottle of champagne in a week or two. Pretty simple.

Here's another example. George is a nice guy, successful at his job and popular with his colleagues. But since he moved into his new apartment his temper had been short and he complains of terrible headaches. Let's see why:

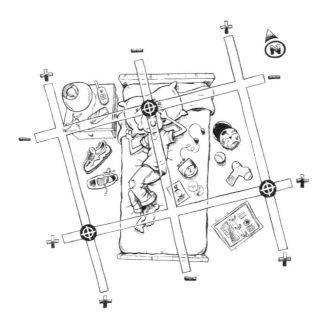

You guessed it. All night George's head is in a Hartmann Knot. No matter what he does to strengthen his energy in the daytime, every night it drains out again because of the harmful vibrations in this spot.

Another factor that contributes to George's headache is the presence of electromagnetic fields that are emitted from his alarm clock, cell phone charger and bedside lamp. Yes, these things are useful but they should not be placed next to George's head. Do you have a clock, radio, telephone, multi-plug, lamp or other electrical appliance near your head, like George? Move them farther away! Throw away your electric blankets. They produce electro-magnetic fields when you turn them on. Even when they are turned off, the wires in them amplify any disturbing vibrations that may be around you. Down comforters will keep you warmer with none of the side effects (and lower electricity bills, too).

It has not yet been explained if these vibrational walls originate in the earth or if they come from space, pulled in by the earth's gravity and reflected back. Maybe they are caused by the interaction between the earth and cosmic rays. I don't know. I do know the effect they have. Through my experience I found that sometimes when I treated a patient, balancing their energy with acupuncture and correct food and medicinal herbs, doing everything that I know should have made them feel better, they would leave my place feeling great but come back in a day or two with no energy again. We built up their energy by day and they lost it by night. I knew I was giving the right treatment and could see that the energy was much stronger after a treatment, so what was happening? Time and time again, I went to check where the patient spent his time. Guess what I found? That's right. Bad vibes! Move the bed and, voilá, no more energy leaking and the patient's health took a turn for the better. I learned from experience that eliminating harmful vibrations from personal surroundings is a very important piece in the puzzle of total health.

As if a world-wide-web of disturbing vibrations is not enough there are other types of subtle vibrations that are even worse. These include mineral deposits, caves, natural faults in the earth and, most commonly, underground streams, either flowing naturally or in pipes.

This is what happens with underground water: Imagine a river. A river flows. It flows in a particular direction. As the water flows through the pipe (either man made or a natural tunnel) it creates turbulent circulation.

This is how it works in an enclosed system. Make a not of this fact because it is very important information. *Why* is this information so significant? What's going on there? When water moves like this, it creates friction. Friction causes vibrations that travel and expand. To give you an example, think of a stone dropped into a calm pond. The waves travel slowly out from the center, right? Well, these vibrations behave in a similar way only in three dimensions.

Have a look at the following diagrams – you will get a better understanding of how this works.

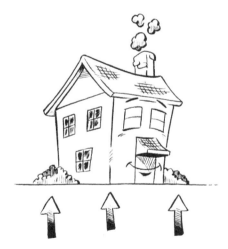

These are normal vibrations of the earth.

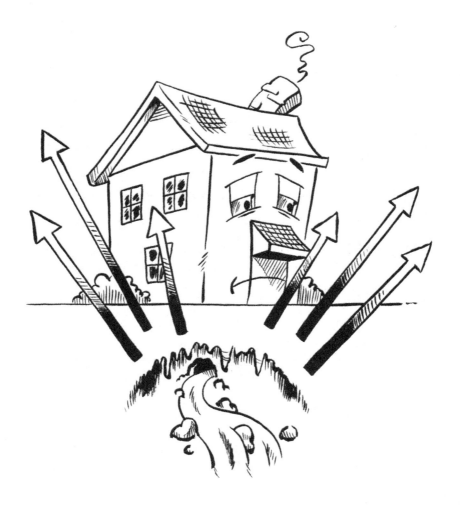

Here's an underground stream. The waves from the running water deviate the normal vibrations causing us to lose our vital connection with Mother Earth.

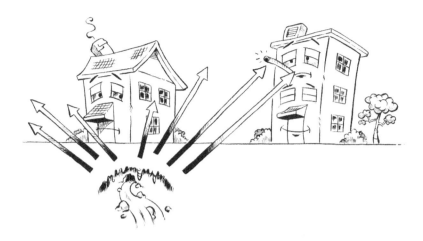

As you can see, that one little stream can affect a wide area.

Look at the apartment house next door. The lower floors are unaffected by the underground stream, but the upper floors catch it!

Some time ago, a friend planned to build a house and asked me to check the lot of him. At the time, he was using the piece of land to graze horses. I found an underground stream running right through the place he planned to build his house. I asked the man who tended the horses where they liked to spend their time; if they liked the shady place near their watering trough. He told me, "Oh, no. They come and drink and then go over there." He indicated another area on the far side of the property. The trough was fed by a spring. The area around it was influenced by an underground stream that disturbed the horses.

Like the horses, experienced dowsers are sensitive to subtle vibrations and are able to locate the presence of underground water. It's great to find water for a well or for irrigation but it's not so good to build a house above an underground stream. What happens? You know that your body is about 70% water, right? The strong vibrations caused by movement of the underground water affect the water in your body. Your own personal water starts to feel a connection with the outside vibrations. Imagine you hear loud music playing. Your foot starts tapping in time to the rhythm. You can't help it. The water in your body can't help it either. These vibrations are great for the underground water but not for your water. When you want to have a good night's sleep the water in your body is busy partying. How do you know if your bed is over underground vibrations? Easy. You continually wake up feeling tired, like you've been partying all night, too.

Just to make things worse, if you live or work in a tall building that has a lot of metal re-enforcement in it guess what happens? The metal in the structure of the building amplifies all vibrations and you get a double dose.

A friend of mine lives in a big house with four bedrooms and a lovely view of the sea. Both she and her son were feeling low so I offered to give them a checkup at their home. When I stepped into the house I felt very uncomfortable. I sensed a slight pressure in my head when I walked in the door. Through my research and experience I have become more aware of and sensitive to the presence of vibrations. My friend has three big dogs. She told me that all the dogs slept in one corner of the house. It was funny to see three large dogs curled up together in one corner. When I checked the house for underground vibrations I found that the only good spot in the house was that one corner where the dogs slept. So, watch your dogs. Their bodies react to the presence of vibrations the in a similar way to ours. They naturally go to the places that are good for us. Draw the line, though, at sleeping in the doghouse.

In the past when people lived closer to nature they knew these things. They would watch the animals and birds and learn from them. People were nomadic and followed animals. They watched where the animals liked to hang out and then pitch their tents there. Today, we suffer because we have forgotten this knowledge.

So, what to do? First of all, if you are not getting a good night's sleep, *move your bed*. With a little practice with dowsing rods or the muscle test (see Extras – Page135) you can find out where the harmful spots are. Ideally, it's best to be in a clear spot with your head to the north and your feet south following the flow of the earth's magnetic field. Second best is with your head to the east and feet to the west. That way you will be aligned with the rotational force of the earth. However, it's better to be any-which-way in a spot that is clear of disturbing vibrations then correctly aligned in a harmful spot.

Watch your plants. Most plants do not like places with strong vibrations. They cannot be healthy if they are exposed to them. More than likely, a person with a green thumb is someone who lives in a place that is not affected by harmful vibrations.

If there is nowhere to move your bed, there are some things that you can do to protect yourself. I'll get to that later in the next chapter.

Another important source of disturbance is electromagnetic fields. Many creatures depend on the natural geomagnetic fields that they use as pathways to guide them on their seasonal migrations. Birds have a center in their brains that responds to magnetic fields. The magnetic field varies in intensity depending on the seasons and the time of day. This is Cosmic Law and all organisms are a part of it - including us. All living beings respond to natural electromagnetic fields to help them to survive. Humans do, too, but we've forgotten how it works.

Over the last century there have been incredible technological developments: electricity, radio, television, household appliances, microwave ovens, personal computers, smart phones, and so forth. All these things create new fields that are different in frequency from those in nature, both in quality and quantity.

What effect do these electromagnet fields have on the body? Imagine a health body as orchestra with all the parts, the organs and the cells playing together in the same rhythm and producing a harmonious sound. Now imagine a loud drum outside the concert hall beating at a different rhythm. After a while, the weakest member of the orchestra will pick up the rhythm of the drum. This player throws off the whole orchestra and pretty soon the sound is no longer harmonious.

A healthy body tries to keep its own rhythm - optimum health - but if it is continually exposed to harmful vibrations in the environment, it cannot stick to its own rhythm and slowly looses the game on all levels. It is very important to understand the duration, quality and quantity of exposure to harmful electromagnetic fields.

What to do? If you have high voltage power lines running above your house or if you live close to a power plant or transformer then *move*. If you have lamps, clocks, extension cords, televisions or radios near your bed *move them*. Just do it. As you can imagine, spending many hours in front of a computer is not so good for you. Make sure that you sit a good distance from the screen and take frequent breaks to stretch and get some fresh air to revive your energy. Protect yourself with an electromagnetic field neutralizer or put an amethyst cluster between you and the computer. I'll tell you why in the next chapter.

7 Rock and Roll

Now, I'd like to tell you some interesting things about rocks. Well, not exactly rocks...This chapter is about crystals, gemstones and magnets and how you can use them to improve your health and well-being.

They say a diamond is a girl's best friend. Why? Why do you think diamonds are prized beyond any other stone? Maybe ancient people knew more than we give them credit for. It has to do with light. A diamond is so precious because all the colors of the spectrum are contained in it.

Light works in a funny way. Sun light contains all the colors of the rainbow. A rainbow happens simply because water vapor in the air breaks light up into its parts. Do you remember the seven colors of the rainbow? They are red, orange, yellow, green, blue, indigo and violet. Together these colors make white light.

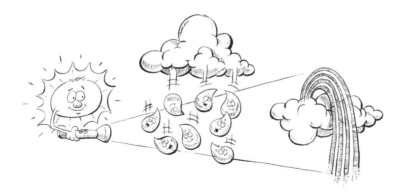

It's very pretty, but what does this have to do with my health? To be healthy is to be whole, to be complete, to have all your systems working optimally together. It's like white light - a total whole spectrum in balance with itself.

We see different colors because each one is vibrating at a different frequency. Parts of us vibrate at different frequencies, too. The trick for having good health is to get our whole body to vibrate in *harmony*. The subtle forms of healing like aromatherapy, flower essences, sound and color therapy all work to increase our life force and bring our bodies into optimum balance. Once we are balanced on the etheric level, good health can begin to come to the physical level, too.

Acupuncture works somewhere in between the physical and etheric bodies. It regulates the flow of energy in the body to increase vitality. Using hair-fine needles to stimulate particular points along energetic highways and byways, acupuncture strengthens and balances the life force, which in turn allows the body's own natural healing to occur. That's why acupuncture has no negative side effects; the body heals itself.

We talked before about balancing the Yin and Yang energy in your body. We saw how all the organs are interdependent. Now I'll show you another system that has only recently been brought to the attention of the West, although it has been common knowledge in Eastern cultures for thousands of years

Do you know about your Chakras? The word comes from India, but each body has seven major chakras. Each is a center of energy; a wheel of light spinning like a whirlpool. They are outward projections of your state of health. Each one relates to a different aspect of your physical, emotional and mental well-being. Each one is also associated with a color and a particular organ. You can think of Yin and Yang in terms of black and white. Now I want to introduce you to the colors.

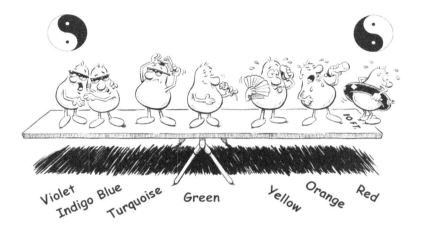

Within the rainbow there are two main divisions of color, the warm colors of the red spectrum (Yang) and the cool colors of the blue spectrum (Yin). All colors are represented in the human body; the warm colors lower down and the cool colors up above with green, the color of nature, right in the middle.

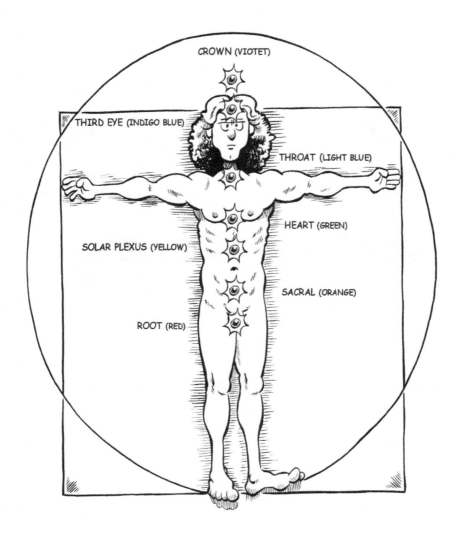

CROWN (VIOTET)

THIRD EYE (INDIGO BLUE)

THROAT (LIGHT BLUE)

HEART (GREEN)

SOLAR PLEXUS (YELLOW)

SACRAL (ORANGE)

ROOT (RED)

The First Chakra (Root) is at the base of your spine. It relates to your life force, survival, strength and power. Its color is red and its gemstones are ruby, jasper and coral.

The Second Chakra (Sacral) is in the center of your abdomen, about a hand's width below your navel. It relates to physical energy, sexuality, romantic and your reproductive organs. Its color is orange and its gemstones are carnelian, tiger-eye and amber.

The Third Chakra (Solar Plexus) is just above your navel. It relates to digestion, mental functions and control of the physical body. Its color is yellow and its gemstones are citrine and yellow topaz.

The Fourth Chakra (Heart) is in the center of your chest. It relates to emotions, feelings and the functions of the heart and lungs, circulation and respiration. Its color is green and its gemstones are emerald, jade and malachite.

The Fifth Chakra (Throat) is at your throat. It relates to communication and expression. It's connected to the tongue, larynx, pharynx and thyroid gland. Its color is light blue and its gemstones are turquoise, lapis lazuli and sapphire.

The Sixth Chakra (Third Eye) is in the center of your forehead. It relates to intuition and perception. It is connected to the pineal gland and to your senses of sight, smell and hearing. Its color is indigo and its gemstones are sapphire, blue agate and aquamarine.

The Seventh Chakra (Crown) is on the top of your head. It is your connection to the Divine. Its color is violet and its gemstone is amethyst.

I'm presenting this very basic information about chakras so that I can go on and give you some practical tips about using stones. There are many good books that can give you detailed information about the chakras. Have a look at the bibliography at the end of this book.

Stones are your friends

One of the most user-friendly stones that I've discovered is the quartz crystal. Quartz is related to the diamond in that they are both colorless (since they are, in essence, all colors) and carry the full spectrum of vibrations of light. Place a diamond or a quartz crystal in the sun and you can see all the colors of the rainbow. The clearer the stone, the brighter the colors. Quartz crystals are either clear or cloudy. The clear ones carry Yang energy and the cloudy ones carry Yin energy. You can use pieces of quartz to help get yourself in balance.

For example, if you are feeling low (Yin), hold or wear a clear quartz crystal or meditate while looking at one. You can also put a clear quartz crystal in a glass of spring water. Leave it there over night. In the morning, remove the stone and drink the water. The presence of the clear quartz crystal "Yangizes" the water and you will feel revitalized if you continually drink "crystallized" water over a period of two to three weeks. Don't drink it at bedtime, though. It might keep you awake.

Here is a little secret for people who love to drink wine but don't like the way they feel the morning after. Place a clear quartz crystal (about the size of your thumb) in your wine before you drink it. Leave it in for about three to five minutes for a glass of wine, or about twenty minutes for a bottle. Not only will the wine taste much mellower but you will not feel such strong effects. Why? We saw before that alcohol is Yin. By bringing it in contact with a Yang stone the extreme Yin is brought into balance, moving closer to the center of the seesaw. This gives a whole new meaning to a drink "on the rocks".

I've done exhaustive research on this subject and have enjoyed every delicious moment of it. One of my favorite experiments is to pour one glass of wine from the bottle, put a crystal in the remainder, and wait a while. I offer a glass of the "crystal" wine to my friends and ask them to compare it to the "control" glass that I poured earlier. I experimented on a friend who considers himself a wine connoisseur. He took the first glass, the "crystal wine". Carefully, he swirled it around in the glass and delicately sniffed its bouquet. Tasting it, he proclaimed, "A delightful little wine... Full bodied and mellow, with just a hint of blackcurrant." I gave him the second glass, the control glass. "You don't expect me to drink this!" I loved the look on his face when I told him that it was the same wine. To this day I'm not sure he believed me. Don't take my word that this works - try it yourself.

The ancient people knew this trick. They placed amethyst crystals in their wine barrels. After some time, the amethyst moderated the strong Yin energy of the wine and mellowed it. In fact, "amethyst" is a Greek word that literally means, "not intoxicated".

Another revitalizing technique is to get two quartz crystals, one clear and one cloudy. Men and women have to do this exercise differently. Let me explain: A human is like a magnet with two poles. In a man, energy spirals from the sky towards the earth: in a woman, energy spirals up from the earth to the sky.

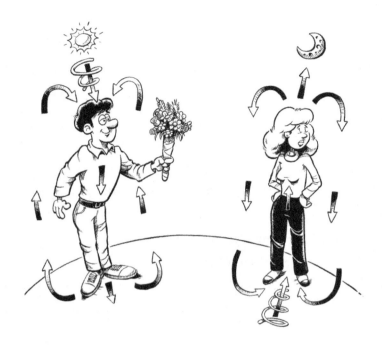

Now the exercise:

Sit comfortably. Make sure that you are not wearing tight clothing or shoes. Remove your jewelry. Ladies first: Hold the clear quartz in your left hand with its point facing away from you. Hold the cloudy stone in your right hand with the point facing towards you. Gentlemen, you hold the stones the opposite way. Hold the clear stone in your right hand with the point facing outward and the cloudy stone in your left hand with the point facing towards you. You'll be able to feel a light electrical current passing through your arms, heart and shoulders. This little current can accelerate your energy flow and help dissolve blockages in your system. Try it and see. I find that it also intensifies my meditation.

Have you ever given any thought to why Kings and Queens of old wore jeweled crowns? To make them seem taller and more imposing? Maybe. But could there be another reason? Rulers need a clear head to make decisions that are a matter of life or death to their people, or themselves. The metal of their crowns and the use of precious stones supported their subtle energy. Their energetic flow was stimulated and their power of perception sharpened. The Old Testament of the Bible gives very specific instructions for making a jeweled breastplate for Aaron, the brother of Moses. (Exodus 28:17-21). There is a legend that Alexander the Great's conquest of the world was halted after he received a gift of a jeweled crown from the existing rulers of a province in India. I believe that the crown was specially designed to cause the devastating headache that lead to Alexander's demise.

Many books have been written about the healing properties of crystals and gemstones. Again I'll ask you to have a look at the bibliography. I promised a simple book so I'll just give you a few more tried and true tips about our friends from the mineral kingdom.

Feel a sore throat (a Yang problem) coming on? Try a turquoise (a Yin stone). Turquoise is a light blue stone. It relates to the Throat Chakra. You can hang a turquoise on a short chain so that it rests in the little hollow at the base of your neck; or tape a small stone there with medical tape. If you do this at the first sign of a sore throat, chances are you won't have a second sign.

For menstrual cramps or indigestion (Yin problems) try taping a carnelian (a Yang stone) to your tummy. A carnelian is a slightly translucent orange colored stone. I know it looks strange but the energy of the stone supports and balances your second chakra which will make you feel a whole lot better.

On a summer day (Yang), when you're feeling hot already, it's better not to wear gold jewelry or amber (they are also Yang). Wearing these will make you feel warmer. Wear them when it is cold to warm you up. Silver (Yin) has the opposite effect.

An amethyst will help protect you from the effects of strong vibrations in your environment. Wear one next to your body for protection. It's a good idea to place an amethyst cluster between you and your computer so that the energy of the stone strengthens your subtle energy making it less vulnerable to the harmful effects of the strong electromagnetic vibrations coming out of the computer.

If you identified disturbing vibrations under your bed or workplace and it isn't possible to move them, you can put amethyst clusters or slices of agate (4-5 inches in diameter) underneath your bed or the chair you work in to dissipate strong underground vibrations. In the case of your bed you will need enough stones to protect its entire area. The stones must be placed under the mattress in such a way that there are no energetic gaps. One amethyst cluster about the size of your fist will protect about two square feet of space. A single bed will need about three stones. If there is space left unprotected the vibrations may be concentrated in one area of your body.

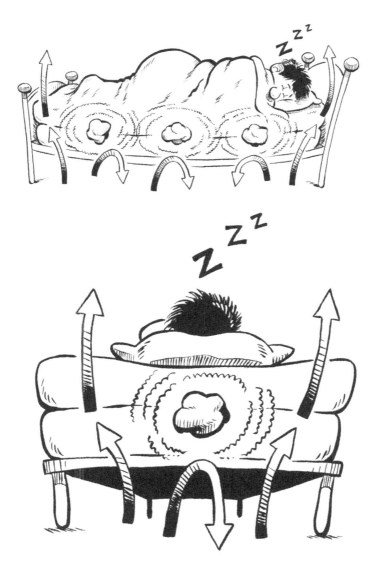

You've got it all covered

To make sure you've got it all covered, sit on the bed and try the muscle test. (see Extras – Page135 for detailed instructions)

Getting back to where we started: a diamond will strengthen and protect your entire aura. So, a diamond really can be seen as a girl's best friend - and a boy's, too.

We have discussed a stone that is full of light, the diamond; now let's now have a look at a very dark one, a loadstone, more commonly known as a magnet. Do you remember playing with magnets as a child? I do. I was fascinated when they together and stuck to one another for no apparent reason. I turned one around and felt them pushing each other apart, but no matter how hard and long I tried, I couldn't push them together. Why not? What was this invisible force that pulled the magnets together or kept apart? Why and what again!

The mysterious force is magnetism. The earth, as I mentioned before, is a huge magnet. Each small magnet works in the same way as it does. Each individual magnet has its own north and south poles. The north pole pushes out and the south pole pulls in. When two magnets are near one another and can move freely their North and South poles will naturally join together. But try to put the two North poles or the two South poles together. Not only will they refuse to stick together, they will push each other apart. Why? In the case of two North (pushing out) poles their force pushes each other apart. In the case of the South (pulling in) poles each one's energy is contracted, there is nothing for the other to pull. The moral of this story: Opposites attract!

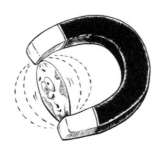

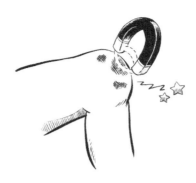

Of all the wonders of the mineral kingdom, magnets are unique. They are the only stones that have their own electromagnet charge. Within their structure they have both positive and negatively charged particles (Yin and Yang). In each individual magnet, the charge flows in one direction, from one end to the other. When it meets another magnet, it will turn itself in such a way that the flow will continue into its neighbor. For two to be drawn together it is necessary to have a force that attracts and a force that repels.

No matter how hard we try to connect similar ends together those invisible but powerful energy won't let us do it.

In a healthy body there is a dynamic balance of positive and negative particles. Through our everyday activities we use an uneven amount of them. Every cell in your body needs to replace the particles that have been used up in order to regain its balance and do its job. That's where magnets come in. Using magnets as a therapeutic tool supports our busy cells and makes us feel good. The stones I mentioned earlier in this chapter work gently to balance your mental and emotional energy, allowing your physical body to heal itself. A magnet's energy works from the opposite direction, penetrating and stimulating the physical body directly, supporting tissues, fluids and organs on the cellular level and speeding the healing process. Once your body feels better, you relax and your mind and emotions become more balanced as well.

Magnets are being used more and more to diagnose and treat diseases. Magnetic Resonance Imaging (MRI) has made it possible to see inside the human body in a way that was not possible in the past. Magnets are used in some delicate surgeries. Experienced magneto-therapists successfully treat acute and chronic diseases as diverse as asthma, paralysis and even cancer in its early stages.

There are many magnetic products on the market. These magnets are not original loadstones but man-made material that has the same magnetic properties. These products are handy to have around. Magnetic insoles can give you a lift. A magnetic mattress can help with insomnia. Therapeutic magnets placed next to injuries will help them heal. Even refrigerator magnets can make bruises disappear faster.

Magnets are particularly effective to treat rheumatism, which is the result of an excess of Yin, an accumulation of cold in the joints and muscles. There is a lack of circulation and a blockage in the free flow of energy, which causes pain and sometimes swelling. Magnets, correctly applied to the joints, work to unblock the stagnant energy and promote circulation allowing fresh blood to carry the accumulated toxins away. I'll explain more about how your internal energy works in the next chapter.

8 Say "CHEE"

Chi (pronounced "chee"), ki, prana - many different names for the same thing: life force. Chi is the life force that flows through your body like a river, all the time, from the moment you are conceived until your last cell dies. The existence of Chi is only now beginning to be known and accepted in the Western world. Oriental martial arts were introduced to the West few decades ago. Martial arts work by strengthening a person's chi. "Chi" is in the name of many styles of Martial Arts - "Chi Gong", "Tai Chi", "Aikido", and so forth. They also train a person to achieve greater sensitivity to the energy both inside them and around them. In that way, practitioners are able to anticipate their opponent's move as if "by magic" and take action before the blow reaches them.

Acupuncture works with the flow of chi in your body. Imagine a river flowing freely to the sea. Picture a busy little beaver building a dam in its stream. The water cannot flow down to the valley as before and the plants that flourished there start to wither and die. The chi flow in your body works the same way. If your chi is blocked, then the life force is prevented from flowing freely and after some time, physical symptoms will begin to appear in your body. That's why acupuncture works so well as a preventative treatment. It relieves the blockages in your energy flow and opens the circulation of your life-force before physical symptoms appear.

Imagine two batteries. One has been in your transistor radio for a few months. Your radio does not play as well as it should. It picks up static and the volume won't go very high. You know it's time to change the battery. You get a fresh one, toss the packet and get ready change it. You open your radio and take out the old battery and put it on the table. The batteries are now lying side by side. The phone rings. It's your Aunt Maude wanting to tell you all about her last operation. You listen patiently, wish her a speedy recovery, and go back to the task at hand. Now, which is the new battery? They look just the same. The only way you can tell which is which is to put one in the radio and see what happens.

Your body works the same way. Your energy "battery" could be running very low but your body would look fine. Maybe your "volume" is down. "I'm not feeling myself today", is a common comment from a person whose battery is running low. What if you leave the spent battery in your radio? If you forget it there for a year or so? You would open your radio and find corrosion or leaking battery juice. Again, the same thing happens in your body. If your battery is left to get weaker and weaker, then eventually you will also see the damage in the form of physical symptoms.

The majority of people on this planet know about the existence of chi, life force. For people raised in Western culture, however, chi is a strange notion; a matter of belief rather than knowledge. People in the West are beginning to recognize that acupuncture works, but, because they were raised in the Western system, they try to find an explanation through that system to justify their observation that acupuncture and other forms of alternative medicine work. That is like trying to find English words in a Chinese text. You can't. If you explain how it works through the Chinese system then it makes perfect sense. (as do many other natural occurrences that baffle the Western trained mind.)

My mother-in-law's dentist told her, "I don't believe in acupuncture." I had to smile when she said told me this. To me it's like hearing somebody say, "I don't believe in gravity". Not so long ago the majority of people in our culture knew the world was flat and that the sun and all the planets revolved around the earth. The few people who believed otherwise and had the courage (or audacity) to say so got into *big trouble!*

As technology developed and broadened our vision (the invention of the telescope, for instance) our cultural norms changed. Now, everybody knows that the earth is round. What else have we learned lately about the earth? What about the science of Ecology? Ecology was a word that most of our parents never heard when they were growing up. Now every school child can tell you what it means. There is a cultural awareness about the necessity to preserve the planet by realizing the impact that separate things have on the whole.

Let's consider, for a moment, our "personal ecology". Imagine that your body is the earth. Around the earth is a protective layer called "the atmosphere". Your body has the same thing. It is called an "aura" or "etheric body". Just as pollutants produced on the earth can create a hole in its atmosphere, so a weakness in your system (caused by internal factors like stress, emotional upsets or an improper diet or external influences such as exposure to strong underground vibrations, or electromagnetic vibration from your television, computers or cell phones) can cause a hole in your protective shield. The hole itself is not the problem. It's what can come in through the hole that can do the damage. In the case of the earth it's harmful cosmic rays, UV rays, or x-rays. In the case of your body, it's viruses and bacteria, which are always around us. Why is it that some people are affected by them and others are not? Ever wondered?

If you would like to experience the chi flow in your body try this simple exercise:

Sit or stand comfortably. Take a deep breath to calm yourself. With your elbows close to your sides, hold your forearms so that they are parallel to the floor. Turn your palms to face one another. Take another deep breath. Keep breathing deeply while you *slowly* bring your palms together. When your palms are about two inches apart, make *slow* circular movements as if you were washing your hands, keeping your palms flat and facing one another. Don't let your hands touch one another; keep them about two inches apart. Feel what's happening. Don't continue reading. Try it!

Did you do it? What did you feel? When your palms got about 6 to 8 inches apart you probably started to feel a slight pulsing. It's important to keep breathing because breath and Chi work together. As you made the circles did you feel a tingling in your palms? What you felt was chi. That's it.

Think about this: Modern Western medicine has been around for about two hundred years - tops. Chinese medicine has been around about 4000 years. Modern Western medicine, with its technological aids like microscopes, scanners, machines that breathe for you and all the other medical wonders, is very good for putting you back together when you are broken. Developments in the fields of molecular biology and immunology have wiped out many previously fatal diseases saving many lives. However, when it comes to quality of health and preventative medicine, the Western way is off the mark. It denies the very existence of the parts of your body that are crucial to your vitality - your chi and your aura.

Time and again I hear stories of people going to the doctor complaining that they "don't feel right". The doctor checks them the "modern" way, finds nothing wrong and either sends them home with a "Tisk, tisk, it's all in your head" or with some medication to calm them so they don't notice that they are not feeling right. Most likely these patients have recognized a blockage in their chi. If their chi is strengthened at this stage, it's likely that a more serious problem will be avoided and the day to day quality of their lives will be greatly improved, as well as their energy levels.

When I was studying in China a doctor told me, "In the West when you go to a doctor, they ask you about your family history. "Did your parents suffer from any particular disease, for example?" Here in China often the patients ask me, "Is your family healthy? Are *you* in good health?" If I can't keep myself and my family in good health why should a person put his life in my hands."

Your good health is in your hands.

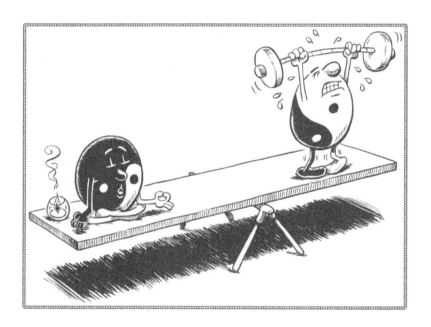

9 The Mysterious World of Energy Medicine

I spoke in an earlier chapter about the unseen vibrations in our environment that have a significant influence on our health and wellbeing. Now I'd like to explain a little more about why this is so and how our body is more than just meat and bones.

When we look at something; this book, a computer, a banana, our own arm – it seems as though it is a solid thing. We use our five senses to perceive our world. We see something, smell it, hear it, taste it and touch it and we know it is real. But what about a thought or an emotion? They are very real, but not something that you can experience with your five senses.

In physics, we learn that everything is in motion. The slower the motion, the more dense the substance. Think of water. In its slowest state of motion it is solid ice. Add some heat; the motion increases and you have a pool of water. Add more heat and soon the water disappears as steam. It's still there, but you can't see it anymore.

We can consider that our body is like ice; it appears to be solid but what we can see is not the totality of who we are. We reflect the image of our Mother Earth. We live on her crust. Deep down inside are layers of soil, stone, molten rock and fire. Above her surface is the atmosphere. Without this subtle, *invisible* atmosphere, life would not be possible.

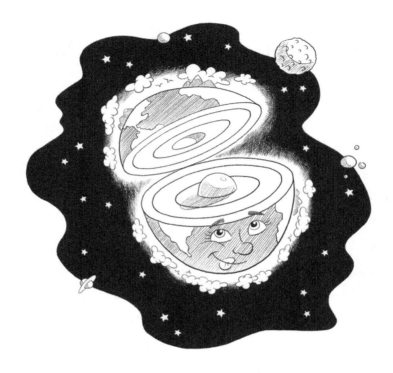

We can experience our physical body through our five senses. Sensitive people and new technologies can access our subtle bodies - thoughts and emotions - the "atmosphere" around us.

In the fifteenth century, Leonardo da Vinci and other proto scientists, delved into the workings of the human body by cutting up cadavers and looking inside. There was much to learn in this way, although a living body works differently from a dead one!

With this knowledge, we were able to observe the anatomical connections within the body on the physical level. Over the years, technologies were developed that extended our senses. The invention of the microscope let us look deeper into the physical body, as did the more recent technological developments such as chemical lab tests, X-rays, CAT scans, ultrasound and so forth.

All these technologies focus on the physical level of our body. These tools were used to see what is going on, but did not provide enough information to explain all the functions that were observed. We began to understand the normal functioning of the body; breathing, digestion, metabolism, circulation, all the visible, observable functions. The development of bio-chemistry provided tests, such as blood counts and urine analysis, to observe and explain deeper functions including the workings of hormones. However, Western medicine cannot explain thoughts and emotions within these, observable, parameters. Yet, these are an important part of us, vibrating on more subtle frequencies than our physical body and have a great impact on its state of health.

Think about the different levels at which we can observe the human body: the physical body, organs, tissue, cells, molecules, atoms, and beyond that – what? The crazy and wonderful world of quantum mechanics! I will not go into details about that here, but I would like to say that ancient cultures have known about the subatomic world and used that knowledge for healing. Since the beginning of the last century science and technology has been developed that enables us to observe and dance with this mysterious level of existence. An understanding how the subtle movement of subatomic particles work is a key to accessing the invisible factors of thoughts, memory and emotions, which are the root causes of many diseases.

To understand how disease starts, picture an empty bucket. Imagine the bucket filling up with things that cause stress to our bodies: wrong food, environmental toxins, tobacco, bad habits, worries, radiation, emotional stress, family stress, stress from our work, and so forth. All of these things build up in the bucket, but nothing is visible until the bucket is full. Something will be the last drop in a full bucket! I could be a tense word, a cold wind, a sleepless night; something not very serious in itself, but on top off all the other things that have been building up it is the one that will cause the bucket to overflow. When that happens, physical symptoms appear.

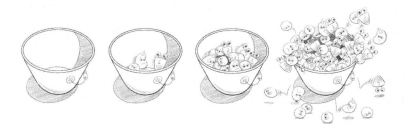

If you simple treat the symptom, the bucket is still full so the next small stressor that comes along will cause it to overflow again, creating a new symptom. Unfortunately, Western medicine is focused on symptoms that can be clinically observed and measured, but does not take into account what is in the bucket – the deeper, built up causes of the disease.

Using energy medicine, I can observe both the physical symptoms and also what is in the bucket. In this way, we get a much bigger picture, inside and outside, visible and invisible. I can see into the bucket before it overflows, addressing a condition *before* it manifests in the physical body. *Prevention is the highest form of medicine.*

When I treat my patients, I help them to slowly empty their bucket by identifying the stressors and educating them about what they can do to prevent them from filling up the bucket again. By working together with cooperation, understanding and consciousness I help my patients change their lifestyle habits resulting in a healthier and happier life!

10 P.S. I Love You

Remember our friends the fish? Now that you have an understanding of the basic idea of this sign, I'd like to explain in a little more detail about what it means.

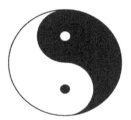

Do you see the one bit of detail on the fishies? Yes, they each have an eye. It is the opposite color from their bodies. This tells us that within Yin there is Yang and vice versa.

In winter (Yin), we occasionally will enjoy a glorious sunny day (Yang). In summer (Yang), there are sometimes showers (Yin). Within each side is constant movement from extreme through moderate and to the other extreme until it can't go any farther and comes back again. So, Yin and Yang are always in movement, creating a *dynamic balance*. Imagine the sign rotating around in three dimensions. Beautiful, isn't it? It's the dance of life.

An example of the principle in action is the effect that alcohol has on the human body. Alcohol, as you remember, has Yin energy. When we have one drink we feel relaxed and in a good mood. Relaxed is a Yin state. If we continue to drink, our tongues begin to loosen. We want to find someone to talk to. This phase is beginning to get Yang. It's getting more outgoing, as are we. Yet another drink brings us to a very Yang stage. Depending on our personality, this takes the form of good-natured, (though possibly out of tune| singing, dancing on the tables, outrageous jokes or even a fight. The morning after all this partying the Yin really takes effect. We want to stay in bed, in the dark with no loud noises.

Another example of Yin and Yang from nature is the monthly cycle of the phases of the moon. The full moon, of course, is the most Yang time of the cycle. It has been noted in various studies that more violent crimes are committed at this time. The word *lunatic* comes from *luna* the Latin word for moon. Someone who was crazy was thought to be under the influence of the moon. I explained before how underground water affects the water in our bodies. Knowing how the moon affects the waters of the oceans in the form of tides, it's not difficult to make the connection that our bodies are also affected by the pull of the moon.

A woman's menstrual cycle is about the same length as one full cycle of the moon. Women who live close to nature and are deeply aware of moon phases generally will menstruate during the new moon. Have you noticed that when women live together their menstrual periods often synchronize? This is the most Yin time of the month. In some Native American cultures, the women of the tribe would spend their menstrual days away from their normal duties. They would spend this time together, not engaging in their everyday Yang activities of preparing food and caring for their families. They would walk in nature and collect medicinal herbs or sit quietly together and tap into the Yin, or feminine energy. Afterwards they would share the insights gained at this time with the rest of the tribe. In today's busy world we have lost this deep connection with the feminine, magnetic energy. Women, remember this information the next time you get annoyed with "the curse"; use this time consciously to tap into your body's deeper wisdom.

Another familiar example is water. As ice it is in its extreme point of Yin. In its liquid form it is at the point of equilibrium – its natural state. As steam it is at its most Yang – expanded and without form.

Consider a seed: Yin, quiet, self-contained. Add energy in the form of nutrients from the earth and heat from the sun, and it begins on its journey toward Yang. It grows to maturity, the most extreme Yang moment of its life cycle. Then it begins the process of returning to the earth, eventually changing back to Ying and losing its form as a plant; its parts being broken up and recycled back into the earth.

The same goes for us. As children, we are growing with Yang energy. We are active and moving all the time. We need more fuel to help our bodies energize and grow. As we reach maturity, we are at the peak of mental and physical activity. As we age, we become more Yin in nature: calmer, contemplative and, hopefully, wiser, having learned from experiences throughout our life. Take your age into consideration when thinking about which foods are best for you to eat.

Once you are familiar with which foods are Yin and which are Yang, start to think about what happens when you cook them. Preparing food is how we bring it closer to balance. Take frozen vegetables, for example. They are in an extreme state of Yin - there is no movement, no bacteria can grow, no decay takes place. Fire is an extreme Yang state. Something will burn until there is nothing left but ashes – and ashes are Yin. We've come full circle.

When you cook meat you make it even more Yang. It crosses the extreme point and when it cools down, is less Yang then before it was cooked. Amazing. Extreme Yin foods are moderated by being warmed up. On a winter's day, to make a meal more Yang, you can use salt, soy sauce or hot spices. To balance a meal towards the Yin side, add more fresh vegetables, either raw or lightly cooked. If you understand the logic it's easy to remember what to eat.

If spicy food is Yang, then why is it that it many places with a hot (Yang) climates traditionally use lots of spices? Mexican food uses chili and cumin. Indian cuisine incorporates curry, chili, cardamom and many other spices. Szechwan food can knock your socks off. Don't the spices and the hot climate tip the balance to the Yang side? A closer look will show that some hot climates are also very humid. Humidity creates dampness in the body, a Yin condition. The Yang energy of the spices counteracts the dampness.

Also, the extreme Yang of spices in addition to hot weather raises people's body temperature, stimulating the immune system and preventing the development of any microorganisms that breed like wildfire in hot and humid conditions. In these countries it is also a tradition to have a siesta after meals. A little nap provides the necessary Yin balance.

If you ever get confused you can't go wrong if you eat everything in *moderation.*

In Chapters Six and Seven I talked about vibrations. This is a *huge* subject. I would like to mention just one more thing that you might have experienced yourself. When you meet a person for the first time, do you sometimes feel really comfortable with that person or sometimes take an instant dislike to them? It has to do with a difference between your vibrational field and theirs. There is a resonance or disharmony between your two energetic fields. Sometimes you may feel uncomfortable in a certain place, or a certain position in a room. The reason is the same – a disharmony between you and the vibrational frequency of your environment. Learn to notice these things. The more sensitive you get to the vibrations around you, the more aware you become of the huge amount of information that is available for the taking if only you know where to look for it.

Now I'd like to say a word about nutritional supplements. It seems to me that every year there is a new "fashionable" vitamin, mineral, combination supplement or "wonder drug" of the herbal world. Certain supplements are useful when you have identified an imbalance in your body and are actively involved in a method of treating this imbalance. but *a supplement is not a substitute* for the nutrients found in food. I always tell my patients that supplements are "secondhand health."You don't want to be secondhand healthy, do you? To become dependent on supplements is yet another "quick fix" and will not lead to long term health and balance. Often, mineral supplements are extremely Yin and will themselves cause your body to be out of

Superfoods are another story. They are nature's gift: living things that give life and are especially useful in our modern urban lifestyle. Some superfoods that I recommend are bee pollen, spirulina, algae from the sea, wheatgrass and wheatgrass juice. These foods support and enhance a balanced diet.

To change the subject… what is pain? Pain is your body's natural way of letting you know that something is wrong. When a child first touches a flame she gets a burn. She learns very quickly not to touch it again. Through experience, we learn to avoid contact with things that cause us pain. This happens on the emotional level, as well. Often, a person who has been hurt in a relationship will hold back and limit his feelings the next time. Once bitten, twice shy. As we begin to understand ourselves, our bodies and our emotions, we can begin to free ourselves of the limitations caused by the experience of pain. To simply *know* that pain is a warning sign whose function is to protect you, not an enemy to be conquered, is an important key.

As we start to find our balance and make friends with our bodies, whole new worlds of understanding and happiness will begin to unfold. Welcome to the adventure of a lifetime.

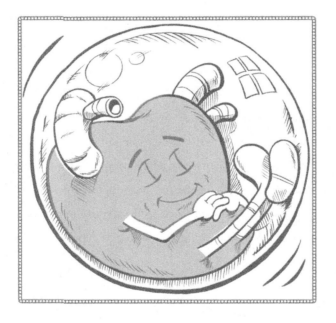

11 What About Gluten?

In 2010 and 2011 I had the pleasure and challenge of working with a compatriot of mine, a world-class athlete. I had seen him playing on television. Although he played well, he had frequent health issues that kept him from fulfilling his full potential. I knew that I could help him and set about arranging a meeting through mutual acquaintances. One of the first things I discovered when I began to work with him was that he had an intolerance to the gluten found in wheat and other grain products. Since he really wanted to be able to play his best he immediately cut all gluten products from his diet. After a few months, his game noticeably improved. His breathing and stamina were much stronger and his health much more stable. The next season he won several major tournaments and the press was talking about "Gluten"!

So, by popular request, here is a simple story about Gluten – what it is and what it does to your insides.

Gluten is a particular mixture of two proteins that exists in wheat, a staple food in the Western world. It's hard to avoid wheat. We enjoy toast, pancakes and wheat based cereals for breakfast, sandwiches and croutons in our salads for lunch, yummy pizza and pasta for dinner…the list goes on!

But people have flourished on this diet for centuries, you may say. Yes, but the quality of wheat was different. Since the middle of the 20th century, wheat has been modified, first by selective breeding and later by genetic modification to ease and increase production. More grain was produced but it was not the same grain that people had been digesting for millennia. The hybrid grain contained substances that our intestines were not designed to digest.

In my medical practice over the past ten years, I have observed that one out of every four or five of my patients had sensitivity, over-reactivity or an allergy to wheat. That is a high percentage of people who are sensitive to a very common food.

Gluten is like glue. It sticks to the lining of our small intestines and interferes with the normal absorption of nutrients from the food we eat. Our intestines are lined with mucus membranes that act as a filter allowing only the tiniest of nutrient particles to pass through and enter our blood stream to be used to fuel our body. Gluten compromises the mucus membranes, leaving gaps through which larger and undigested particles can pass into our bloodstream.

Your body is very smart! It recognizes that these larger particles do not belong there. Naturally, there is an immune reaction as your body sends out the troops to defend itself against the perceived invaders. The immediate result is an inflammation of the intestines.

If gluten in continually consumed, the walls of the small intestines thicken and do not allow even the good little nutrients to be absorbed. This condition leads to a variety of symptoms such as bloating, gas, diarrhea and cramps.

Since our life-blood flows throughout our body, undigested particles in the bloodstream can wreak havoc all though our system. In previous chapters I told you how, according to Chinese medicine, there is a correlation between various organs. In this case, it is important to remember that the small intestines are paired with the heart. The heart is the filter of emotions. An emotional imbalance or disturbance can further upset an already compromised small intestine.

The partner of the large intestines is the lungs. If there is excess mucus in the large intestine, chances are there will be excess mucus in the lungs, as well. The creation of excess mucus is the body's way to cleanse itself and get rid of what it perceives as toxins. Excess mucus compromises breathing through limiting the amount of oxygen that can be absorbed, and can also block the nose, adding to the strangulation! It's an uncomfortable condition to be in, but our body is just doing its job and trying to protect us!

In Western medicine, an increase of mucus in the respiratory system in combination with psycho-emotional problems can look like respiratory, asthmatic or sinus problems. Since Western medicine addresses the symptoms rather than holistically understanding the cause, these conditions are viewed as something they are not, because the root cause is not understood and often treated in ways that don't work and can cause further problems over time.

As you may have guessed by now, the root cause of these conditions is often the over consumption of gluten.

In Chapter 9k, I presented the example of a bucket of toxins that slowly fills until it overflows, resulting in visible symptoms. If someone is in good shape, sometimes the body can handle the gluten experience for a while. But, in the long run, consuming gluten products on a daily basis will fill up the bucket resulting in the symptoms of allergy.

These symptoms vary depending on the sensitivity of the individual, the amount of gluten consumed, the level of stress and the many other factors mentioned earlier in this book the make up the puzzle pieces of optimal health.

A person with a mild case will feel discomfort in his or her tummy and bloating after meals. The most extreme case is known as "Celiac Disease", where there is extensive damage in both the large and small intestines preventing proper digestion. The intestines lose their ability to distinguish between beneficial and harmful particles. There is constant inflammation and often malnutrition. A person will eat, but the nutrients cannot get where they need to go.

Be aware that gluten is not the *only* culprit here! As I said before – fast food = fast death! Food is not a game. Do not watch television while eating or as in the case of more and more young people, do not play violent or exciting computer games while eating. Do not eat standing up. Make mealtimes sacred! Say grace! Give thanks! These traditional practices serve a very practical purpose – they reduce stress and help us focus on the meal we are about to consume thus aiding healthy digestion.

Digestion is directed by our autonomic nervous system, which controls the normal function of hormones, enzymes, neurotransmitters, normal metabolism and biochemistry. If we input excitement, for example bad news on television, violent programs, computer games, and so on, while we eat, the autonomic nervous system reacts to the unconscious fear and anxiety and digestion is no longer a priority.

Besides gluten, similar processes happen with over consumption of dairy products and sugar. When symptoms appear, people go for allergy tests and are tested with thousands of substances, but the main point is lost! Most of the time, the cause of the allergic reaction is a weakness in the intestine walls caused by the most common foods that we eat! Compromised intestines compromise our immune system. Often there is constant inflammation, fatigue as the body fights night and day to remove the inappropriate substances in the bloodstream, causing constant stress. With the immune system barking up the wrong tree, as it were, the door is open for all sorts of pathogens, funguses and so forth. Not a pretty picture!

So, what to do? Give your tummy a holiday! Cut out all wheat and other products that contain gluten for one month and the see how you feel. The good news is that intestinal walls can and will repair themselves quickly when they are not compromised by disturbing factors.

During this month, make an effort to reduce stress in your life. Make time to meditate or walk in the park; make time for yourself and relax a bit every day. Once your intestines are back in balance, the occasional piece of toast or pizza is fine to eat – *just don't stress over it!*

I am very happy that, through my work with the athlete, there is a much great awareness of gluten and how limiting its consumption can really benefit your health. Knowledge is power; but knowing is not enough. Apply what you have read in this little book and you will see the difference it will make in your health and wellbeing.

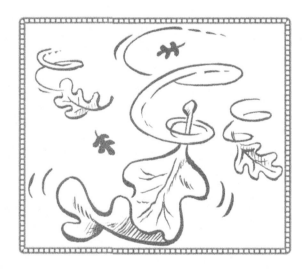

12 The End of the Beginning

You now have a greater understanding of your bodies, both physical and etheric and how they interact with your environment.

Your body is your greatest teacher and healer. If you learn to quiet your mind, let go of all the advertising hype and listen to the wisdom of your body it's simple to be healthy.

Now that you know that your health depends on many things and that, although popping a pill may make you feel better for a while *true and lasting health depends on you taking responsibility for your body.* That's what this book is about. *your responsibility!*

Where do you start to make the change? You already have, my friends, by reading this book. You now have all the information and tools that you need to take another step on the road to good health.

Think about the food that you put into your body. Consider the weather and your level of activity. Eat fresh foods that are in season where you live. You'll know what's in season by the price. Fruit and vegetables that are in season are cheaper. If your current eating habits are a long way from ideal, slowly start to make changes. It may take some time to change the foods that you've been eating and enjoying for years so don't feel you have to do it all at once. Start out by avoiding extreme foods and eating more of the things that are closer to the center of the seesaw.

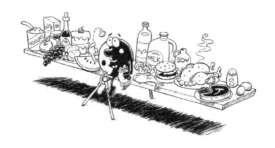

It's okay to *occasionally* eat something you really enjoy but that you know is not particularly good for you, but don't keep unhealthy food in your home – *simply do not buy it*! Let's say you feel a craving for a donut; ask yourself, "Do I really want this *now*?" (The key word here is *now*.) If you can wait, then don't eat it. There are plenty of donuts in the world. If you *really*, *really* want one, then you can go and get one. Get out of the habit of eating things just because they are there without asking you body if it really wants it. It's that simple...

Avoid processed foods. In affluent countries, people often have more money than time. A whole industry exists to provide "convenience" food to save the cook time and effort. But pay attention to the ingredients on the package of this "food". The list of ingredient often reads more like a chemistry book than a cookbook. Some companies are now beginning to make products with fewer additives and preservatives, but the only way to really know what you are eating is to make it yourself. Buy the freshest and least processed foods you can. Organic foods produced without the use of pesticides or hormones or genetic modification are the best. They may seem more expensive, but in the long run they are cost effective. You get better quality food - more nutrients for the same quantity of food. You will eat less because your body will get the nutrition it needs. In addition, if you don't buy convenience foods you'll find your shopping bills actually go down and, if you are on the heavy side, your weight will probably go down, too.

If you wake up feeling tired every morning move your bed. Ask a friend to help you use the Muscle Test (see Extras – Page135) to find a better spot for it. Leave it in the new place for ten days to two weeks. If you are still waking up feeling tired, move your bed again. If you cannot move it, then get some stones as mentioned in Chapter Seven and put them under your mattress in order to protect yourself against the disturbing vibrations. Once you find a place where you can sleep well *make sure you sleep enough*. Give your body a chance to renew and rebuild itself during your hours of sleep.

Be aware of electromagnetic fields (EMF's) in your environment. Move all electrical equipment away from your bed. Check the other side of the wall near the head of your bed. If there is a fuse box, circuit breaker, computer or microwave oven, *move your bed*. When working on a computer, take frequent breaks for fresh air. Look into devices that neutralize the effects of harmful environmental vibrations.

Learn to relax and take it easy. Watch your body when strong emotions threaten to push you off balance. *Remember to breathe.*

Get more oxygen into your blood by walking in nature; walk in unspoiled rural areas if you can, or in a park. Listen to the birds. Find a sport, dance class or any physical activity that you enjoy and participate on a regular basis.

Drink pure spring water. Sometimes tap water contains chemicals that can be harmful to your system. It's better to drink pure spring water whenever you can. It's inexpensive and often tastes much better!

Find things you like to do and do them. If you are in a job that you hate, think about changing jobs or find an aspect of it that you enjoy and try to get in a position where you will spend more of your time doing that. If you can't change jobs then make time for a hobby that really gives you pleasure. If you can't think of anything you'd like to do, think back to what you enjoyed as a child: model making, playing with trains or dolls, climbing trees. You can still make models, collect trains or start a doll hospital to repair a child's treasure. If tree climbing is your thing, remember that you may be a little heavier now then you were a decade or two ago, so choose a tree with strong branches. You know you've found something you love doing when hours pass without you realizing it.

Turn off the television. Or better still, don't turn it on. If the first thing that you do when you get up in the morning is to turn on the television, get out of that habit. Find a radio channel that plays music you like. Avoid news-only and talk channels and listen to music stations - you'll still get enough news and traffic to know what you need to know. Better yet, listen to a favorite MP3, CD or enjoy silence. When you listen to the news and advertisements, be discerning. Don't believe everything you hear, and don't let the information avalanche throw you off balance.

Spend time with people you like. And I don't mean only sitting around a television set. Get to know other people. Go out and play together. Go for walks or join in sporting or social events. Spend your time with positive people and with the kind of people you would like to be yourself. If your current situation means you have to spend time with people whose company you don't enjoy you may have to make some changes. As you get healthier, you might find people you thought were friends resenting the fact that you are developing yourself. You may seem too independent and they may feel that you no longer need them for support now that you are taking responsibility for yourself. These people are not *real* friends. A real friend wishes the best for you. As you become healthier, you will meet others who are walking the same road - a road that, down the line, leads to a much happier life. You will see that the journey itself is the exciting part - the things you learn, the people you meet, the fun you have on the way - not just the eventual destination.

Life is a dynamic exchange of Yin and Yang. Sometimes we have good days, sometimes bad days and some days are right in the middle. Bad days are our teachers. They give us an opportunity to see what is not working in our life. Once we are aware of what it is, we can do something to change it. As you make the necessary changes, you will find the bad days will become fewer and the bad things that happen are not really *so* bad. Be patient.

When we have a good day, we can share our happiness and energy with others. A kind act or even the sight of a smiling face can start a pleasant chain reaction in the world that can have consequences beyond imagination.

Fill your emotion quota with happiness and share it with others. The more you give, the more you will get back.

Bon voyage and happy trails!

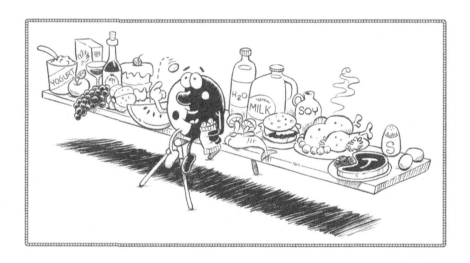

In the Kitchen

I have suggested that one way of balance is through your stomach. Besides understand the principles of Yin and Yang, I want you also to consider the act of preparing and eating your food. If you cook or eat in a rush, you lose many of the benefits of your food. Why? In a word, *stress*. Our busy, contemporary lifestyles create stress and worry that affect the stomach, whose job it is to separate "impure" energy from "pure" energy; that is, the nutrients from the waste products. If you want to get the most from your food, take your time preparing and eating it; connect yourself with your "fuel."

Before you prepare a meal, set you cooking "stage". Make your kitchen a pleasant place to be. Keep it clean, tidy and free of clutter. Have some flowers of herbs growing by the window. Put on some music that you enjoy. When you cut your vegetables, think about how they grew from a tiny seed into something delicious and nourishing. If you cook meat, thank the animal for providing for your nourishment. Balance your mind, body and spirit as you cook. Infuse your ingredients with happiness – singing in the kitchen makes everything taste better. Don't take my word for it. Try it and see.

As I mentioned before, when you eat, don't watch television or read the newspaper. Focus on the food you eat and on the good company you are sharing it with.

Here are some simple and delicious recipes that not only please the palate but the nose and eyes as well.

Donna Marijana's Magic Soup – *Serves 4*

In the land of my birth, we always have soup as our first course with lunch. Here is the basic recipe:

1/2 large onion, minced

1 large carrot, grated

1/2 cup uncooked rice

1 tablespoon vegetable oil

1 stock cube* & 5 cups filtered water (or 5cups of homemade stock)

1/2 cup peas, chopped mushrooms or celery (in addition to or instead of the rice) –optional

Sauté the onions in the oil over a medium high heat.

When they dry out and become translucent add the carrots and cook for a few minutes more.

Add the water and the crumbled stock cube (or the stock). Bring to the boil. Add rice and vegetables and simmer until they becomes soft, about 10-15 minutes.

Season with freshly ground black pepper, a little dill or chopped parsley. To make the soup a little more Yang, add soy sauce. To make it a little more Yin, add a small amount of vinegar.

This soup is particularly good for you at the time of year when the seasons change. It supports your stomach and spleen and keeps your digestive system in good condition.

The Famous 3-2-1 Combo

This combination is familiar to all my patients. It is a wonderful blood tonic and superb energizer. If you don't feel well, have a little every day, otherwise once a week is enough. There are two ways to enjoy the benefits of this combination. One is as a salad and the other is as juice. Why 3-2-1? Because you will need:

3 "red" things:	beets, apples, carrots
2 green things:	celery, parsley
1 yellow thing:	a lemon

If you can get home grown or organic vegetables – *do!*

For juice: just put one beet, one apple, one or two carrots, a stalk of celery, a little parsley and half a lemon through your juicer. You can vary the amounts to taste. Sip a glassful after meals.

For a salad: grate the beet, apple and carrots. Chop the celery and the parsley. Use the juice of the lemon to make a dressing with a little olive oil. Garnish with walnuts. The oil helps your body to absorb the vitamins and minerals. Try this at home. It tastes much better than it sounds!

The Chinese say "Satisfy your eyes with colors". Translation: If you eat a variety of foods, something of every color, then your nutritional needs will be met.

If you use on of each item, you will get 2 large glasses of juice or enough salad for 4 servings; feel free to use more of what you like best.

Warning: The first time you drink this juice or at this salad, your body will probably absorb all the nutrients in the beets. However, the second or third time, your body won't need so much and the result will be bright pink liquid waste! Don't panic if you see what looks like blood in the toilet; it's just the excess beet juice being eliminated.

Note from Francesca: I always hated beets. When Igor suggested that I eat them to strengthen my system, at first I thought, "No way". But, slowly, slowly I began to eat cooked beets when I saw them at salad bars. (The first time I ate them I had a cold and couldn't taste anything) Eventually, they didn't seem so bad. The first time I tried them raw, grated in this salad I really liked them. Now I eat them often with real enjoyment - and feel a lot better, too.

~

At the first sign of a cold – or to feel better if you've caught one – try this

Stephanie's Hot Toddy

This is Francesca's mom's family remedy – taken just before going to bed at night it will promote sleep and recovery.

Juice of ½ a lemon
1 teaspoon good quality honey
A good shot of Scotch whiskey
1 cup of hot water

Combine; drink it while it's still hot and sleep well!

Old Fashion Gingersnaps –

Makes about 3 dozen medium sized cookies.

When the winter winds blow and the sky is gray and drizzly, the ginger and cinnamon in these delicious and easy to make cookies will warm you right down to your toes. Make a double batch of dough and keep some in the refrigerator (before you roll it out); pop a few cookies at a time in to oven and fill your kitchen with the soothing smell of home- make goodies.

2 1/4 cup flour (preferably gluten-free!!),

1/2 teaspoon cinnamon

1 teaspoon ground ginger

1/3 cup butter

1/2 cup brown sugar or 1/3 cup honey

1 egg, well beaten

1/2 cup molasses

2 teaspoons baking soda

Preheat the oven to 350° F.

Mix the flour, cinnamon and ginger together.

Cream butter and gradually add the sugar, beating until light. Add beaten egg and molasses.

Dissolve baking soda in 2 teaspoons of hot water and add to the creamed mixture.

Combine the dry ingredients and creamed mixture. Chill.

Roll out on a lightly floured board to 1/8 inch thickness and cut into fun shapes with cookie cutters. Place cookies on a greased baking sheet. Bake in at 350° for 10-12 minutes.

And, last but not least, a soul warming drink from India…..

Chandar's Honey, Lemon & Ginger Drink

For each serving you will need :

About an inch and a half long piece of fresh ginger
The juice of half a lemon
A spoonful of good quality honey

Gently wash the ginger then mash it with something hard (a flat bottomed rock or the side of a wide knife will do the trick!)
Put the ginger in a small pot with a cup of water and bring it to a boil.
Put a spoonful of honey in the bottom of a mug and add the lemon juice.
Add the hot ginger water (straining it so you don't get bits of ginger stuck in your teeth.

Stir well and enjoy.

The World Famous Muscle Test

To do this "test" you will need either a friend or a suitcase that is *almost* too heavy for you to lift (the suitcase has to be heavy, not the friend). It is based on the premise "your body never lies".

Your body can show you which places are affected by harmful waves. You'll be able to detect places affected by underground waves or electromagnetic fields.

Have your friend stand facing you, and extend her right arm straight from the shoulder, parallel with the floor. Tell her to resist the pressure you'll put on her arm. Press down *slowly and evenly* on her forearm while she resists you with all her strength. This is not a contest to see who is stronger, so take it easy! Both you and your friend should be able feel the point where it's difficult to resist the pressure.

Maybe you won't be able to push her arm down at all! I have a friend who is a professional body builder. I tried the test on him. In a place that was not affected by harmful waves, I could practically do chin-ups on his out-stretched arm. Then we went to quiet corner of his gym, an area where nobody liked to work. I had checked the space before and knew that it was influenced by an underground stream. We tried the test there. You should have seen his face when I pressed his arm down with two fingers. It's sad to see a grown man cry!

If you can easily push down your friend's arm, move to another spot; the first one might not be "clear". If you are much stronger, ask your friend to push your arm while you resist. Once you've established the amount of resistance in a clear spot, it's time to try it in an area where there are harmful waves. Have your friend stand with her back to a television set. Try the test with the set turned on and also with it turned off and see what happens.

Test the place where you spend a lot of time: your desk, your television chair, and the most important place of all, your bed. Move the bed out of the way and do the muscle test where your head would be, and then all the way down to your feet. If your resistance is low, *move your bed!* Find a spot where your arm stays strong.

If you can't find a friend to try this, do it by yourself. Fill a suitcase to the point that you can just about hold it in one hand when your arm is extended out to one side of your body at shoulder height. Move around the space you want to check; if you can hold it without discomfort, then the place is good. If it is too heavy to lift, then the place is not good for you. Don't do this test too many times in a row; your arm may get sore.

You can do this same test with other things, too. Test a cell phone, tobacco or chocolate and watch what happens. Try a banana or a tomato. Hold the item in question in your left hand, over your heart. Have your friend press as before. You can test different foods, drugs or vitamins to see which ones can help you and which may harm you. Try the same thing on different days. What's bad for you on Monday might be okay on Thursday. Some things are always a no-no. Find out which ones and avoid them. Try this at your next party. The stronger the "victim" the better. Cell phones and cigarettes are always good for a laugh.

Suggested reading

To learn more about how your body works:

The Body Atlas, A Pictorial Guide to the Human Body, Steve Parker, Dorling Kindersley, 1993, <u>London, New York, Stuttgart</u>

How your emotions influence your health:

You Can Heal Your Life, Louise Hay, Hay House, 1984 <u>My edition is from London but it was first published in the States – I'll look in a bookstore when I go.</u>

A good book about Diet:

Eating Your Way to Health, Dietotherapy in Traditional Chinese Medicine, Cai Jingfeng, Foreign Language Press, 1988 , <u>Beijing</u>

A very good resource for educational information on all sorts of conditions:

Healthy Healing, A Guide to Self Healing for Everyone, Linda Rector Page, N.D., Ph.D., Healthy Healing Publications, 1997

To learn more about your chakras:

Hands of Light, A Guide to Healing Through the Human Energy Field, Barbara Ann Brennan, Bantam Books, 1987, <u>New York</u>

Some good books about the healing properties of Crystals and Gemstones:

The Power of Gems and Crystals, Soozi Holbeche, Piatkus, London, 1989

Focus on Crystals, Edmund Harold, Ballantine Books, 1987, <u>New York</u>

Healing with Crystals and Gemstones, Daya Sarai Chocron, Samuel Weiser, Inc., 1988, <u>York Beach, Maine – Chocron is the last name</u>

Everything you ever wanted to know about Vibrational Medicine:

Vibrational Medicine, New Choices of Healing Ourselves, Richard Gerber, M.D., Bear & Company, <u>1988, Santa Fe, NM</u>

Mind openers:

Anatomy of the Spirit. Caroline Myss, Ph.D, Harmony,1997

The Biology of Belief: Unleashing the Power of Conciousness, Matter and Miracles, Bruce H. Lipton, Hay House Inc,. 2011

Inspiration:

The Four Agreements: Practical Guide to Personal Freedom, Don Miguel Ruiz, Amber-Allen Publishing ,U.S. 1997

Selected Bibliography

Beinfield,Harriet, L.Ac. and Korngold, Efram, L.AC., O.M.D., *Between Heaven And Earth, A Guide to Chinese Medicine,*_Ballantine Books, New York, 1992

Becker, Robert O., M.D, *Cross Currents, The Promise of Electromedicine,* Penguin Putnam, Inc. New York, 1990

Becker, Robert O., M.D., and Selden, Gary, *The Body Electric: Electromagnetism and The Foundation of Life,* Quill, William Morrow, New York, 1985

Kuan, Dr. Hin, Chinese Massage and Acupressure, Berg Publishing, Inc. New York, 1991

Lu, Henry C., *Chinese Foods For Longevity, The Art of Long Life,* Sterling Publishing Company, Inc., New York, 1990

Michio Kushi, *Your Face Never Lies,* Avery Publishing Group, Inc. New Jersey, 1983

Thurnel-Read, Jane, *Geopathic Stress: How Earth Energies Affect Our Lives,* Element Books Ltd. Great Britain, 1995

Made in the USA
Las Vegas, NV
06 May 2025

21831284R00085